WALTER T. HUC

From WALES *to* PNEUMOCYSTIS *and* AIDS

Centuries of Serendipity

From Wales to Pneumocystis and AIDS
Centuries of Serendipity
All Rights Reserved.
Copyright © 2015 Walter T. Hughes, Jr., M. D.
v3.0

Outskirts Press, Inc.
http://www.outskirtspress.com

ISBN: 978-1-4787-5375-9

Outskirts Press and the "OP" logo are trademarks belonging to
Outskirts Press, Inc.

PRINTED IN THE UNITED STATES OF AMERICA

outskirtspress
DENVER, COLORADO

Foreword

This book is written for my family – my children, grandchildren, siblings and their progeny. I expect the readership to be solely these relatives and perhaps a few friends. Therefore, not striving for literary acclaim and sales promotion I can write as freely as I wish knowing their love and devotion will forgive literary incorrectness. Nevertheless, I am obligated to document accurately facts as I recall and research them.

I began this work soon after the demise of **Jeanette**, my dear sweet wife of 57 years. Now, at 84 years of age, with not much else to do, I have reflected upon my years with humility and with gratitude for the hundreds of people who have contributed to my survival, happiness, family and professional life. At this point I realize most vividly that the greatest reward in my life was to have **Jeanette** and children for whom I have supreme love, pride and joy. **Jeanette** and I were blessed with **Carla Hunt, BS, MS**, a superb Teacher, my constant helper and editor of this manuscript; **Greg Hughes, MS, PhD,** a dedicated Clinical Psychological Counselor, speaker, teacher (U. Memphis) and family comedian; and, **Chris Hughes, M.D.**, a kind and compassionate person in addition to Surgical Director for Liver transplantation, Thomas Starzl Institute, U. Pittsburgh Medical Center.

I have attempted to chronicle many of the details of my life from birth to present day in order to maintain a memory of family and friends, events of my life that occurred by plan and by chance, trivial anecdotes and some philosophical premises I consider important.

I cover several aspects of my professional work for two reasons. First, that's what I do and did; and secondly, to help explain my time away from family when I wanted to be there.

I use the word "serendipity" in the subtitle because I like it; it has a nice ring to it and I don't have to worry about editorial overview in this manuscript. Horace Walpole coined the word in 1754 to mean "a fortunate experience" or "a pleasant surprise." More recent interpretations are "luck that takes the form of finding valuable or pleasant things that were not looked for." I would extend the meaning further to include "a blessing from God."

While in recent years I have written a few novels as historic and non-historic fiction, the pages of this work have no vestige of fiction and all events and characters are real. I have attempted to avoid embellishment of personally favorable events, though subconscious effects cannot always be excluded.

Regrettably, I realize that due to my weakness of memory and my unawareness of many contributions to my welfare from friends, relatives and colleagues, serious omissions will inadvertently occur in this writing. I apologize.

Walter Thompson Hughes, Jr., M.D.

Table of Contents

CHAPTER 1

Wales to Virginia

It has been said that a person with the name Hughes anyplace in the world carries Welsh blood. I believe this to be true. My own Welsh heritage has been well established through documents and handed-down family stories. In younger years I gave almost no attention to Wales and family from the old country. It was a country rarely mentioned in the news, even during the World Wars, and overlooked in Geography 101. However, later in life I developed a keen interest in Wales because of a somewhat serendipitous event.

In July 1988, at age 58 years, I was in England to give a presentation at the annual meeting of The Society of Parasitologists held at the University of Bristol. While there I had arranged to meet separately with some investigators from The Wellcome Research Laboratories at Beckenham, UK, to tell them of some studies I had just completed on one of their drugs in early laboratory development.

Sitting around a cocktail table in the Lounge of the Bristol Hotel, I was able to tell the Wellcome group that my studies in animals had shown their antimalarial compound, yet to have a name, but designated No. 566C80, was highly effective against *Pneumocystis carinii* pneumonia, the major cause of death in patients with the frightening new Acquired Immunodeficiency Syndrome (AIDS). Joy was expressed by all and more will be said about this later.

The day following my talk to the Society I decided to venture out alone in the warm summer day and explore Bristol. In particular I wanted to see the "New House" Chapel built in 1739 by John Wesley, the place where Methodists began. The downtown location and small size of the structure made for a quick visit. I soon came to realize that Bristol was located near the border of England and Wales. So, in the afternoon I travelled by bus into Wales, simply to be able to say that I had been there and with little expectation of much more.

After crossing the Severn Bridge into South Wales near Newport, the bus moved into the countryside toward Swansea. I soon began to experience a feeling of excitement, but not knowing why. This was a very special place. Without any religious connotation, I thought of Wesley's Alders gate experience that caused him to say his "heart was strangely warmed." I became fixed on the landscapes. The green pastures studded with grazing sheep, rolling hills and sloping valleys, large calm lakes with crystal azure water and distant mountain peaks reaching the clouds seemed familiar, as did the cool refreshing climate. I had a feeling of *Déjà vu*, but I did not know for what. I saw almost nothing more of the country due to my need to be back in Bristol for an evening meeting. It was only later when I began to research the country and my heritage that I realized the basis of these feelings, which I'll discuss a little later. In a sense, it was the microbe *Pneumocystis carinii* that serendipitously caused me to find the beautiful country of Wales in the summer of 1988.

Now, dear family and friends let me give you a brief sketch of Wales because most of you probably know less about it than I. Like me, Wales is very old with an established human habitation dating back to the Ice Age more than 10,000 to 12,000 years ago. I have learned that some very old things and very old people like me may fade, dwindle and become overlooked in the modern scheme of things. That's clearly not the case with Wales; in fact, it is just the opposite. Wales has become more beautiful and lovable with age, as have we octogenarians. It might just be that the pristine preservation of Wales today is in part because the Welsh wanted to keep this intriguing place to themselves without intruders.

Wales is a little bitty country with a footprint of only about 8,000 sq. mi; but it is thick and tall, because of mountains. Five mountains in the area of Snowdonia – *Eryri* **(FIG. 1-A)** are more than 3,300 ft. in height; the other 15 Welsh mountains are smaller.

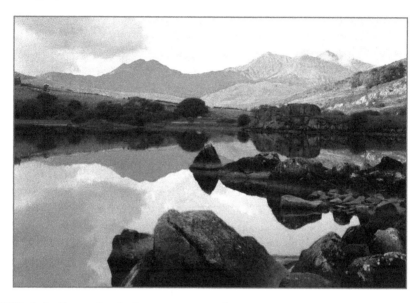

FIG. 1-A: Snowdonia Mountain, Wales (photo Len Green – Fotolia.com)

The country measures 170 miles from north to south and 60 miles from east to west. It is bordered by England on the east and by sea in all other directions providing a very long 730- mile coastline. Also, more than 50 islands, such as the famous resort area of Anglesey, Wales lie in the seas near the coastline **(FIG. 1-B).**

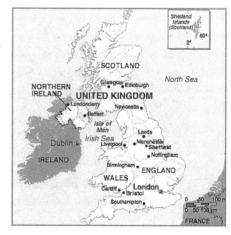

FIG. 1-B: Map of Wales and the United Kingdom

The current population is 3,063,456 people with 96% being White-British and 2.1% non-white. The population is most dense in South Wales in the cities of Cardiff (capitol), Newport and Swansea near the English border. Cardiff is 150 miles from London and 50 miles from Bristol. Some clustering of the population is also found in the northeast area around Wrexham. During and after the Roman Conquest of Wales from 48 AD the rich mineral resources (e.g. gold, copper and lead) of Wales began to be extracted and utilized in metalwork, a factor in my *Déjà vu* experience to mention later.

The weather in Wales is often cloudy, windy and wet with relatively mild but cold winters and warm summers. The Welsh flag displays the legendary "red dragon", symbolic of pride in heritage **(FIG. 1-C)**. Unforgivably, the Welsh drive on the wrong side (left) of the road.

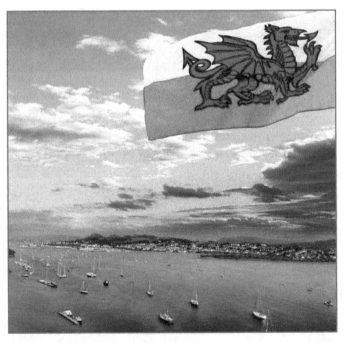

FIG. 1-C: Welsh Flag – "The Red Dragon" on Conway Castle, Wales (Samoff – Fotolia.com)

The name **Hughes** appeared in the Middle Ages (5th century) before much English influence occurred in Wales and when a patronymic system was used for names. People were named after their fathers with no system for last names, so a given name would be followed by "Son of (father's name)." After the Norman Conquest in the 12th century the English system of nomenclature evolved modifying the patronymic system to add an "s" on the end of the father's name in place of "son of." Therefore, the name Hughes indicates that at some time or times in the past relatives had the first name of Hugh. Hugh came from the French name of Hue or Hughe.

Interestingly, engraved in the back of my grandfather's large solid gold pocket watch, now owned by my wealthy brother Joe (I inherited the rusty 1848 Civil War rifle) is his name Josiah L. Hugh_ss_. He lived from 1837 to 1921 and I can find no explanation for this choice of spelling of his name in the 19th-20th centuries, except maybe his will to retain some Welsh history.

A Family Crest or Coat of Arms was often devised by families and clans with pride in heritage in Wales as well as elsewhere. These logos were displayed on armor, flags and buildings. Several images of a 'Hughes' Coat of Arms, varying in design and meaning have been found but with little information to certify one over the other as valid for my branch of the family. An example is shown in **(FIG. 1-D.)**

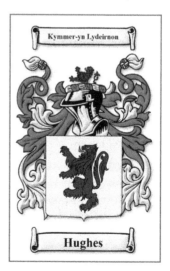

FIG. 1-D:
Hughes Family Crest, Wales

Kymmer-yn Lydeirnon

Hughes

I have not attempted to fetter out the many centuries of Hughes history in Wales. Were I Methuselah my remaining years would not be adequate to write a history of Hugheses in Wales. A case has been made for our descent from Royal princes, several Saints, Bishops and from Roderic the Great. This sort of thing has never interested me because firm supporting data are lacking and, by armchair logic I know that I am descended from Adam and Eve, and no one can top that. And besides, if I really searched diligently I might find a Hughes I would not want to claim. So far they have all been clean.

The 1881 British Census reports the relative frequency of the surname Hughes to be highest on the Welsh island of Anglesey (Yens Mon), some 37 times greater than the British average. Of course the Hugheses would flock to Anglesey!!! From their origins in Wales to present day, the Hugheses have sought the best of the world around them, even despite poverty in some cases. This island off the northwest coast of Wales, now connected to the mainland by bridge is a premier site of the country for natural beauty, tranquility, resort activities and is the residence of Prince William and Princess Catherine after their marriage.

There are many accounts of the immigration of Hugheses from Wales to America, even before there was a United States of America. There is evidence to show that Richard Hughes settled in Virginia and Joshua Hughes in Roxbury, Massachusetts in 1634; and that Griffin and Jo Hughes landed in Virginia in 1635. Joseph Hughes and another Richard Hughes came to Georgia in 1738 and 1744, respectively.

Interestingly, Welsh immigrants or immediate descendants of Welsh immigrants made up the largest ethnic group (16 in all) of signatories of the original draft of the **U. S. Declaration of Independence**. It is noteworthy that Thomas Jefferson's family came to the United States from Snowdonia, Wales. Moreover, George Washington, Abraham Lincoln and Gen. Robert E. Lee were of direct Welsh descent.

My intent is to focus only on the Hughes from Wales that led to my branch of the family in Tennessee. Historians agree that our branch goes back to Hughes brothers who first emigrated from Wales to settle in the colony of Virginia during the early 1700s. Three brothers, Orlando, Leander and William Hughes came to Virginia from Glamorganshire or Caernarvonshire, Wales. Others may have come soon thereafter. At this time Virginia was the most populous English colony in the New World.

Orlando and Leander had land grants in Powhatan and Goochland counties near Richmond in 1740. On March 20, 1743 Orlando's son Leander purchased land in St. James Parish in Goochland County from John Woodson. Soon thereafter, on November 25, 1743 he obtained 390 acres on Pidy Run of Willis River by Patent from the Royal Land Office granted in the name of King George II and signed by William Gooch, Lieutenant Governor of the Colony of Virginia. Two years later Orlando was granted 400 acres on the north branches of Cat Branch of Willis River under the name of King George II. On April 23, 1755 he was awarded another Royal grant of 800 acres.

The Hugheses prospered with land acquisition in Virginia, expanding into Washington and Lee Counties throughout the remainder of the 18th century, after which some began to move westward through the Cumberland Gap into Kentucky, Tennessee, Missouri and elsewhere.

A thorn in the flesh of genealogists, and made more painful by the Hugheses, both in Wales and America, was the common practice of repeating given names from generation to generation, even without designations of Sr., Jr., II, III, or 'son of', 's', etc. Over and over the given names of Orlando, Leander, Josiah, John, William, Thomas, and others are found from the 17th century to now. *In lieu* of modern DNA genotypes, dates of death and birth have served as guides for specific identity.

Our branch of the family stems from **Orlando Hughes**, the brother who originally came from Wales to Virginia in the early 1700s. He had a son Josiah, who in turn had a son **Leander** born on January 1, 1794 in Virginia, who moved to Tennessee and died on May 4, 1868 in Bradley county, Tennessee.

CHAPTER 2

Bradley County and Déjà vu

In 1839 **Leander Hughes** (1794-1868) obtained a tract of land in what became Bradley County, Tennessee. He moved his family from Virginia into a house on a hill **(FIG.2-A),** with peaks of the Blue Ridge Mountains in the far distance. Subsequently, "he and his descendants became large land owners and progressive citizens of the community in which he settled." Throughout the 18th century in Virginia and during the settlement in Bradley County the Hugheses seemed continually poised for opportunities for Land Grants from governments of England and America, as well as other low cost land sales. My contemporary mind would think that these early Hugheses were skilled at grantsmanship and that this skill seems to have diminished in present-day Hughes attributes.

The area in southeast Tennessee to later be designated Bradley County **(FIG. 2-B)** was a part of the Cherokee Nation until May 2, 1836, only three years before Leander Hughes arrived. On this date the Tennessee General Assembly named the 340 square miles extending southwesterly from the Hiwassee River to the Georgia state line as a county named after Col. Edward Bradley, a hero of the American Revolutionary War. Survey of the land began in 1837 and lands were placed on sale with prices based on when the parcels came up for sale. Those properties becoming available during the first four months were priced at $7.50 per acre; the next four months were $5.00; then, $2.00; then $1.00 per acre. Finally, the last was sold in 1841 at one cent per acre.

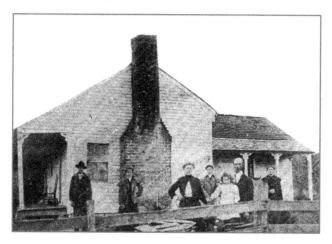

FIG. 2-A: Homestead of Leander Hughes' settlement in Bradley County, Tennessee

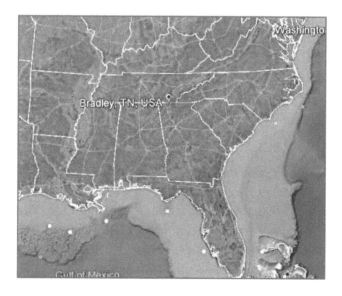

FIG. 2-B: Location of Bradley County, on the Tennessee-Georgia border (Google earth).

At the foothills of the Great Smoky Mountains and not far from the Blue Ridge, Appalachian and Lookout Mountains the terrain of the Hughes land was parallel ridges and valleys. The climate was seasonal with average temperature of about 57 degrees F.; humidity of 76%, light snows in winter and warm summers. The some one thousand acres of the Hughes land bordered north Georgia and was part of an area of vivid historical events.

Once a part of the Cherokee Nation the Bradley County Indians were finally forced to sign over much of their land, first to the British and later to the United States. In 1812 a small town, Charleston, Tennessee about 25 miles from the Hughes farm, in what would later be Bradley County was established as site for the U. S. Agents of Cherokee Affairs, also called the Cherokee Agency and the Hiwassee Agency. It soon became known as the "Gateway to Indian Country." A brother of the Cherokee Chief John Ross had a store at the agency until it closed in 1838.

President Andrew Jackson, elected in 1828 and no friend of the Indian, succeeded in passage of the Indian Removal Act of 1830, calling for the removal of all Indians from their homes and relocation to lands west of the Mississippi River in Oklahoma by 1838, a year before Leander Hughes arrived. Another event spurred on the tragedy. Gold was discovered in Dahlonega, Georgia; about 50 miles from the Hughes homestead, and started the first big gold rush in America. Georgia politicians quickly devised means to redistribute precious Cherokee land to White settlers, and many Cherokees moved across the border into Tennessee to safety.

The Cherokee also inhabited a nearby area in Tennessee called the Copper Basin since the 18th century. A village called Duck town was named after Chief Duck. The U.S. Government took over control of the Copper Basin in 1836 as a part of the Treaty of New Echota. Nuggets of native copper were discovered in 1843 by a prospector, four years after Leander settled on the Hughes place. More than 30 mining companies were operational by 1855. The mining and processing methods resulted in the release of large amounts of sulfur dioxide that killed surrounding vegetation from a weak sulfuric acid rain. To this day these hills remain devoid of vegetation and an adjacent town is called Copperhill, TN.

One of the most devastating and shameful events ever to occur on American soil began in May 1838 here in southeast Tennessee and north Georgia. The U. S. Army, under the command of General Winfield Scott with seven thousand soldiers amassed all Cherokee men, women, children and their limited belongings into collection camps before a forced westward movement. The Indians languished during the summer in these camps until August 28, 1838 when the first group left followed by 12 more groups of about 1,000 Indians per group. The migration was cruel because the Cherokees lacked clothing for cold weather, adequate food, and were exposed to disease. It was said that each campsite along the way became a burial ground marking the trail, famously known as the **"Trail of Tears" or** "Nunna-da-ul-tsun-yi" ("the place where they cried" in their language).

Of the some 14,000 Cherokees on the trail in 1838, 4,000 died from cold, disease and starvation. Overall, with subsequent trips around 100,000 Indians survived the migration on this trail. A main trail crossed Tennessee to Memphis (over 300 miles) and then moved along the Arkansas River to the new lands.

Now, here is another **serendipity ditty.** In 1969, at age 39 yrs., more than 30 years after I lived at the southeast Tennessee Home Place, I moved to Memphis to take a position at a new, small, and unknown hospital named **St. Jude Children's Research Hospital.** It was a two-story building located downtown on a big lot near the Mississippi River and not in the best part of town. It had been built over a somewhat swampy plot once called Gayoso Bayou. But what a marvelous little place it was and I loved it.

I had been at St. Jude a couple of years when one Saturday morning I decided to ride my bright yellow ten-speed Schwinn bike from my home in Hein Park to the hospital. By doing so I noticed an historical marker somewhat overgrown with vines, just inside a back entrance to the hospital. I had never seen or heard about it before. This State of Tennessee Historical marker showed that this site was on the *"Trail of Tears"* and commemorated the suffering of Cherokee Indians trekking from near the Hughes land in southeast Tennessee westward. I have since pondered over what had happened over time on this one square mile or so of the Lord's earth in Memphis, Tennessee, where I have been privileged to live and work. I'll ramble on a little about this because it intrigues me (Old people are allowed to ramble, it humors them).

Long before the arrival of suffering Cherokees across the St. Jude site, the Spaniards trampled along this same area with Hernando Desoto to first view the Mississippi River, where now the huge Hernando Desoto Bridge spans the Mississippi River to Arkansas. They too suffered disease and famine. Because of this mosquito-infested Gayoso Bayou site, epidemics of Yellow Fever often devastated the city of Memphis; once in 1878 reducing the population from 45,000 to 20,000 people within a fortnight, which I write about in *The Yellow Martyrs*.

Importantly, this Yellow Fever epidemic moved U. S. President Rutherford B. Hayes to establish an investigation with recommendations that led to the establishment of the U. S. Public Health Service. Also, an innovative infrastructure in Memphis was created to provide safe drinking water through the use of pumping stations to move fresh water from underground Artesian wells to homes throughout the city. The swamp of Gayoso Bayou was drained and covered providing the base for future buildings on the hallowed one-mile in downtown Memphis. The **Memphis Water Works** became a model known around the world as an important component for healthy infrastructures of cities. It was a major factor in reducing waterborne diseases where people once got their drinking water from the Mississippi River and other contaminated sources. One of the original innovative brick pumping stations was built on this hallowed ground and still exists at St. Jude, as a part of history where a major impact on the health and welfare of people was made.

For a century this ground on which the Cherokee once trod was the site of one of the first and largest hospitals in Memphis, the St. Joseph's General Hospital that provided care to hundreds of thousands of Mid-southerners. It was here that **Rev. Martin Luther King** died after being shot at the nearby Lorraine Motel in 1968. After St. Joseph's Hospital, came St. Frances Hospital on the same site and it was later moved to Memphis suburbs. The now famous St. Jude Children's Research Hospital covers every inch of the square mile and more with over 4,000 employees working to prevent and relieve human suffering. I now think even more of the place as **hallowed ground** with some sort of sacred feature, and I cherish this odd "Trail of Tears" connection to my home place.

I shall spare you here of the lengthy genealogy of Hugheses as to who begat whom in the lineage from Wales to Bradley County Tennessee and refer you to a comprehensive article, entitled "Leaves from the Family Tree" by Penelope Johnson Allen, State Chairman of Genealogical Records, Tennessee Society, Daughters of American Revolution (Compiled by John Morgan Wooten, Historian of Bradley County Tennessee), and published as a special article in *The Chattanooga Times,* March 15, 1936. I focus on this reference because its informational resources are perhaps most valid for the early Hugheses in Tennessee. The several Orlandos, Leanders and Josiahs are found. Sorry, but that's the way it was. I've often wondered why no one throughout the centuries of the Hughes family was ever named Walter except my Dad and me. Should that tell me something?

In brief, as best as I can put it together, Orlando Hughes who immigrated from Wales to Virginia had a son Josiah, who had a son Leander (1794-1868) who moved to Bradley County Tennessee in 1839 and who had a son Josiah L. (1837-1921) who married Martha Smith and had a son, my father, Walter Thompson Hughes, Sr. (1877-1938) who married Millie Collett in 1925. They had 3 children: myself, Walter T. Hughes, Jr. (1930-); my brother, Josiah (Joe) L. Hughes (1933-) and my sister, Katherine M. Hughes (1936-).

You can find the early history of the Hughes family in Bradley County etched in stone in the Sugar Creek Cemetery located a few miles from the home place. **(FIG. 2-C)** shows a photo of a portion of the Hughes plots and the "Hughes Mausoleum", more accurately called a "Grave House". (In a mausoleum interment is above the ground. In a grave house interment is below the ground). The brick and slate structure covers the graves of the family founders in Tennessee, Leander (1794-1868) and Martha Hughes (1797-1876). I believe my father later in life had a role in the building of this grave house because he had a passion for building things and it carries signs of his handiwork. I do know that he built a beautiful gazebo in the cemetery where visitors could sit and rest. It is noteworthy that the organization of churches was given priority by the settlers in this area, beginning during the 1820s to bring Christianity to both Indians and new White settlers. The Methodists were the first denomination in the area, just before the Presbyterians. Also, carefully documented and often mentioned was the location of "The Tavern" kept by Mr. John Cowan.

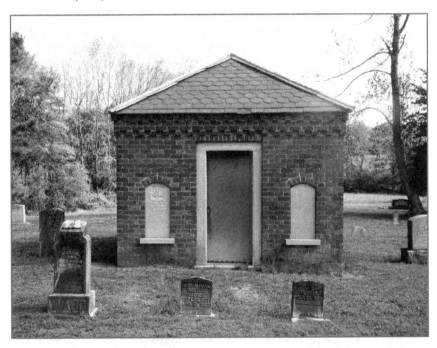

FIG. 2-C: Hughes Grave House at Sugar Creek Cemetery

You may be wondering, as I did, why on earth did Leander Hughes move his family from the populous Colony of Virginia where his ancestors from Wales had prospered for a century, where life was good, and civilization was far advanced beyond that of the western frontier now emerging from east Tennessee and north Georgia in 1839?

You may also be wondering, what caused that big *Déjà vu* experience I had when I first put foot on Welsh soil on that summer afternoon in 1988?

After considerable contemplation I believe I have an explanation for both issues. The magic word is ***DÉJÀ VU***. This stems from the fact that the unique area in the mountainous east Tennessee is now and has been for millennia remarkably similar to the country of Wales. Mount Snowdonia in Wales and the Great Smoky Mountain in Tennessee extend more than 3,000 ft. into and above the clouds and they are terraced with crystal clear lakes and hiking trails; cattle graze the rolling hills and valleys; the climates are similar with crisp fresh air, moderate winters with snow in mountains and pleasant summers. Even the mineral resources of copper and gold are remarkably similar. Despite the fact that I had not been to my Bradley County home for more than 20 years when I entered Wales even briefly, I had feelings from childhood experiences from home. Perhaps Leander had similar feelings of closeness to the land of his fathers.

CHAPTER 3

Home Place

Over the years the Hughes family clustered around the "Home Place" of Leander's original house on the hill. I recall three additional homes on the place built for brothers and cousins and located within sight of Leander's porch. The family's lumber business and hundreds of acres of prime timber were a part of the place including the sawmills, a planing mill, a single room office building and some related structures. Several acres were cleared and cultivated as farmland with barns and stables. A county road leading from the farm was named Home Place Road and joined Spring Place Road leading into the town of Cleveland, TN, about 15 miles away. In more modern times Home Place Road became a state road named Hughes Lake Road (can see on Google earth).

The only image I can find of my birthplace is in **(FIG. 3-A)**. A glimpse of the two-story white house built by my father is seen in the background. It was located on the hilltop and had incorporated a portion of the original 1839 home-place of Leander Hughes **(FIG 2-A)**.

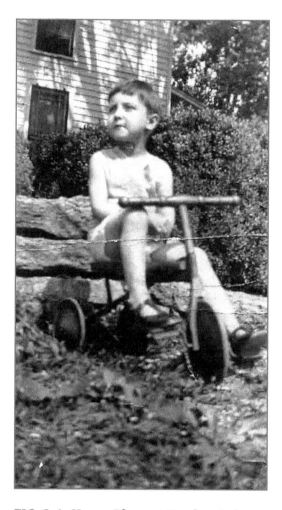

FIG. 3-A: Home Place at Hughes Lake; our House in Background. Walter Jr. on tricycle made by Walter Sr.

It overlooked a lake and the yard was nicely landscaped down the hillside. A white tear-shaped gazebo was in the front yard. I know the tricycle was made by my father and I expect my clothes were made by my mother. As a child and as an adult as well, I had the confidence that my father and mother could do anything.

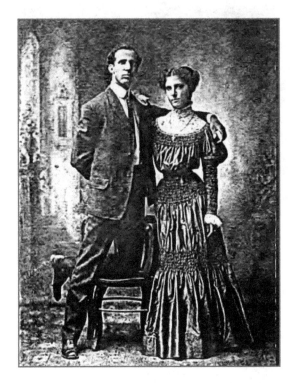

FIG. 3-B: Walter, Sr. (1877- 1938) and sister Amy Hughes

(FIG. 3-B) is my father Walter, Sr. as a young man standing beside his younger sister Amy. She was his favorite sister and he often said so. They had much in common and enjoyed reading and talking together. Unfortunately, Amy died at a young age, as did another sister Susan and brother Amos. An older sister Mollie married James Gregory of Dalton, GA. Her daughter Ruth was active in the Daughters of the American Revolution, married Rob Hamilton, a prominent north Georgia businessman and Mayor of Dalton. Walter's older brother John was associated with him in the lumber business until his demise in 1908.

The photo in (FIG.3-C) shows my father at about 49 to 50 years of age. By this time most of his family had died and he had become the sole proprietor of the family business, the Hughes

Lumber Co. which dated from the settlement of the family in 1839. He was also owner of the "Home Place" of some 1000 acres of heavily timbered land. The lumber company had been successful over the years and was comprised of sawmills and a planing mill that prepared lumber of various sizes and shapes for building things. After selling specially planed lumber to a casket company, he decided he could make caskets as well or better than those in the Cleveland Casket Company (about 15 miles away from the Hughes home place). So, he started the Hughes Casket Company and added another building near the planing mill. My mother helped for a while with the casket linings. I've been told my father and mother would often give free caskets to some of the poor folk in the area. I do remember my mother saying my dad was a "soft touch." He soon realized the casket was not really the end of the line and that considerable profit came from the funeral home. Then, he opened the Hughes Funeral Home on 3315 Broad Street in Cleveland, TN, phone number 716. (How did I remember these numbers at age 84 yrs. when I often forget the dose of penicillin?).

So, at the time of his death in 1938 Walter Sr. was running the Hughes Lumber Co., the Hughes Casket Co. and the Hughes Funeral Home. Despite these ventures he remained fixed as much as possible at the Home Place doing things he liked to do.

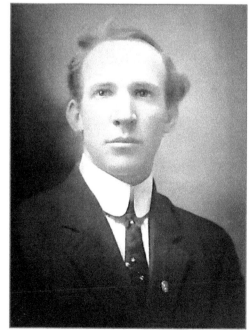

FIG. 3-C:
Walter Hughes, Sr.
at 49-50 yrs. old.

The picture of our mother in **(FIG. 3-D)** was made when she was about 70 years of age. My father had died in 1938 of streptococcal pneumonia – about a year before penicillin became available. I was almost 9 years, Joe was 6 years and Katherine was 3 years old. Our mother as a single mother devoted her entire life to us, often with difficult times and sometimes alone, she persisted and provided us with constant love and attention. Joe, Katherine and I are eternally grateful for her love and devotion.

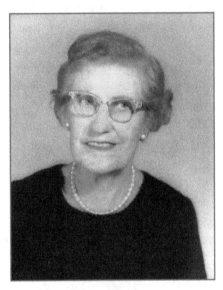

FIG. 3-D: Our mother Millie at about 70 years.

The following is copied from an article in ***The Cleveland Banner*** on October 22, 1938:

"Walter T. Hughes, 61, local mortician, died in a local hospital Friday night of pneumonia which developed following an attack of influenza about ten days ago. He had been kept in an oxygen tent in a desperate attempt to save his life.

"Mr. Hughes was born in Bradley County, the son of Mr. and Mrs. J. L. Hughes, pioneer settlers in Bradley County, on the vast farm in the southeast part of the county that his father bought from the Indians.

He was engaged in lumber and planing mill business for many years and manufactured coffins in a small way which he sold direct to this community and adjoining areas. Four years ago he purchased property on south Broad Street, opening a modern funeral home.

"Beautiful Hughes Lake is situated on the plantation he owned on the Spring Place Road. Surviving are his wife and three children, Walter T., Jr., Joe and Katherine; one sister, Mrs. J.H. Gregory of Dalton, Georgia. Funeral services will be held Sunday at 2:30 at Sugar Creek Church. Pallbearers asked to serve are Darius Felker, Willie Lacy, Robert Clayton, French Collett, Oina Maples and Robert Hamilton."

The picture in **(FIG. 3-E)** is my favorite of my father and mother. I would label it "The real Walter and Millie." It shows them as free spirits at the Home Place on their beloved Hughes Lake. They did what they wanted to do and found almost complete fulfillment of their lives at the Home Place. The photo was taken about 4 or 5 years after they were married and in their favorite play/work clothes. They sit in a boat my father made, floating on the lake he also made. He built a large concrete dam across the drainage of clear water springs and creeks to back up a 7-acre lake of crystal clear water that came to be known as Hughes Lake. As a child I remember this boat. My dad took me for rides in it. I recall it was always as shown, water in the bottom because he was never able to make it watertight. What is not seen is the motor from a Model A Ford automobile that he had installed in the stern? I do remember that in some of our rides, we moved faster with rowing than with the motor. Nevertheless, it must have been one of the first motorboats in Tennessee.

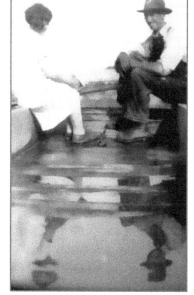

FIG. 3-E:
"The real Walter and Millie"

21

The first six years of my life were spent in the rural "Home Place" in Bradley County, TN, some 15 miles from the nearest town of Cleveland. I was born there on May 16, 1930. Most babies, like myself, at this time were delivered at home by relatives or midwives. I don't recall much about this event but it must have proceeded satisfactorily.

I recall clearly that I was a "Daddy's boy." I was the first child and the only child for three years and spent almost every moment of the day with him. I could go to work with him because most of his day was at the businesses located on the home place near our house. My favorite place was his workshop where he made many exciting things, and I believe his favorite place as well. In the late 1920s he had built a fore bay from his lake to a large waterwheel attached to the end of a building in his plant. The waterwheel turned a generator for electricity to run machines like planers, rip saws, drill presses, band saws and lathes. People came from all around to see Walter's electric plant.

To protect me from the hazards of the shop he brought a child-size casket from the casket shop, cut two large side-by-side holes in the bottom and mounted it on the wall about four feet above his workbench. I was placed into the box with legs and feet dangling below and where I could watch all that was happening in the shop but could not escape from my perch. I recall only one vivid problem to my happy day. In his tedious work my father wore reading glasses. I desperately wanted reading glasses like his. On a trip into Cleveland he took me to the 5 and 10 cent store to buy me some reading glasses. Only tinted sunglasses were available. I must have spent hours in my box with soap, water and a washcloth trying to remove the dark lenses to look like my dad's glasses.

Electricity from his generator was far ahead of its time in rural Tennessee. He had rigged our house and a ring of incandescent lights around a portion of the lake. People from distances in the county and nearby Georgia came to see the lights and swim in the lake eventually to become known as Hughes Lake.

My life has been blessed with wonderful siblings: my brother Joe three years younger and my sister Katherine, six years younger than myself. In childhood Katherine was the pretty, cheerful, smart and lovable one. Joe was funny and entertained the family. Unfortunately, I lacked these attributes.

When I was about 7 years old our mother went into Cleveland for shopping. She surprised Joe and me with Indian suits that she expected to be met with joy. I was joyful but Joe was not. Stores in Cleveland often were limited in stock. They only had 2 Indian suits, so I got the largest one and Joe got the smallest **(FIG.3-F)**. To say the least Joe threw a fit. He was upset because his hat had fewer feathers than mine, his jacket and hat had fewer ornaments than mine; my outfit was called "Chief" and his was called "Scout"; and besides, his pants were way too long.

When our parents took us to Stanfield Studio in Cleveland for the picture (I suppose they thought we were cute) Joe absolutely refused to have his picture made. Finally, I was able to hold him

by the arm for the photo to be snapped **(FIG.3-F)**. Later in life, probably while he was in medical school, Joe learned about the middle child syndrome and concluded it applied to him. He in turned passed the concept (humorously) on to my middle child Greg who to this day refers to it when it comes to his advantage.

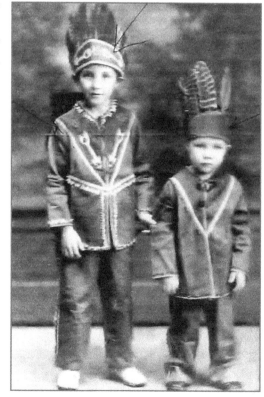

**FIG. 3-F:
Walter and brother Joe
in Indian Suits**

During my days on the farm at the Home Place my father, mother and I would often go "into town" on Saturdays for shopping. My mother's sister, Lora Lacy and family lived on a large farm about halfway between the Home Place and Cleveland on Spring Place Road.

We always, without exception, stopped for a visit to my dear "Aunt Lorry" because she always had something good to eat on the kitchen table and I could always go to her well in the backyard, dip a long-handled gourd into a bucket of cool sweet water for a drink. She was a precious person we all loved. She had a daughter China, and two sons, Hayden and Jasper. Each of her children excelled. China became a school teacher throughout her life, Hayden became an important farmer in Bradley County and Jasper became a successful business man in Cleveland. Interestingly, Jasper's son Allen Lacy became the overall C.E.O. of Sears Co. with offices in Chicago. Another favorite and lovable aunt was my mother's sister Tressa Clayton. She and her husband Robert along with my mother's only brother French Collett and a sister Leola Wrinkle did more than other relatives to help my now single mother to raise her three young children. My mother's sister Clara Felker was financially well off in Cleveland and her only child Estes Felker became a successful Pediatric Surgeon.

CHAPTER 4

Cleveland and Arnold Memorial School

When I was about 6 years old our parents decided they should move "into town" to provide us access to a good education. Cleveland had a sound public education system recognized with high marks. Arnold Memorial School was progressive and clearly the best of some five city schools. So my dad moved us to a place near this school, about one mile away. Pre-school and kindergarten programs were nonexistent at this time, so I began school at age 7 years in the first grade at Arnold Memorial School.

As I reflect on my education in elementary school, high school, college and medical school I realize clearly that the most important were the years of early elementary education at Arnold Memorial School. In support of this stance I can still (at age 84 yrs.) recall the names of my teachers. Miss Bunny Kate taught first grade. Others included Miss Mildred Blevins, Miss Kate McClellan, Miss Mamie Thomas and Miss Lillian Duff. All were dedicated teachers and all were referred to as "Miss..." in keeping with southern tradition and as means to designate respect. I expect the budget for the school system in this small town of some 15,000 people in southeast Tennessee in the 1930s did not exceed payment for meager salaries and building maintenance. Nevertheless, in some way, a simplistic educational program was more successful than many present-day big city school programs and served us well. One example comes to mind – the Music Memory Contest.

The Music Memory Contest was held during the second semester of the seventh grade and was the device of Miss Lillian Duff. Each Friday afternoon during the cold winter days an hour was devoted to preparation for the contest to be held during the last week of the school year. Promptly at 1:00 pm the ritual began. Miss Duff, smile-less with a physical profile like Beethoven, removed the cover from an upright Victrola in the corner of the classroom, brought from her home, and opened the lid to show the spotless turntable and the funnel-shaped speaker. At the side a crank wound up the system after which she donned white cotton gloves to protect the precious record as she removed it from the protective sleeve and placed it carefully on the turntable. Then began the music - Brahms, Mozart, Beethoven, Schubert, Chopin, and others. As the music played she wrote a biography of the composer on the blackboard and students copied it into their spiral-ring notebooks. Neatness counted. Pieces were played over and over and Friday after and Friday. On the big day, "The Music Memory Contest," held on the last week of the school year, students were poised at desks with tablets and sharpened yellow No. 2 pencils. Miss Duff would play a few measures of a classical piece and we students wrote the name of the musical rendition and also a brief biography of the composer. Tablets and notebooks were turned in and at the closing ceremony of the school year the winner was announced. The winner had a gold foil star pasted on his or her notebook. This was a prestigious award among the students. I did not win but I did receive a book, *Biographies of 100 Composers,* from Miss Duff. This book, coated in clear polyvinyl for preservation, still resides more than 75 years later on a bedside table in my home.

I mention the Music Memory Contest because it introduced me, a Tennessee country boy, and many students like me, to the pleasures of classical music which I have cherished and cultivated all my life. Importantly, in present times of expensive and complicated educational systems, is to point out the simplicity and efficacy of this educational tool, developed, executed and paid for by a dedicated teacher in rural Tennessee.

On other occasions, teachers lined Arnold eighth graders double-file along the sidewalk and marched us a mile or so to a small college, named Bob Jones College, located on Ocoee Street in Cleveland. This college emphasized two topics, *The Holy Bible* and Shakespeare. The Shakespearean plays we were privileged to attend were in our minds vivid performances by the college students in colorful dress among impressive scenery. They made exciting and indelible memories to our young minds. Again, these events cost nothing but the time, efforts and imagination of our teachers. Later the college moved from Cleveland to Greenville, South Carolina to grow to the nationally recognized Bob Jones University. The site on Ocoee Street is now occupied by Lee University.

I don't recall much in the way of sports events at the relatively new and progressive Arnold Memorial School, except maybe the times we boys organized among ourselves on the playground after school. Buddies would choose teams for baseball or football, depending on the kind of ball we could come up with at the time. As teams were chosen I recall I was usually one of the last to be chosen because I was not very good in managing any kind of ball. I was never, then and for the rest of my life, very interested in sports participation. I have often regretted that early on I did not develop athletic skills. Later in life I tried golf and tennis but could never appreciate the joy of grown men spending much of their lives trying to hit a ball into a hole in the ground or across a net. One problem I had with after-school playground activities was to make sure my cumbersome "horn case" was in a safe place where it would not be forgotten to be carried home.

Sometime during the seventh grade another "freebee" was offered at Arnold Memorial School. The Music and Band Director at the high school we would soon be attending, came to Arnold School once a week, after school hours, to help interested students to learn to play a musical instrument. I remember clearly my first encounter with the locally well-known Bradley High School music teacher and band director. I thought Mr. Mountain was well named; he was a short man with girth about the size of his height. He examined my hands, pressed my lips with his fingers and told me I had attributes for playing the trumpet. This satisfied me because I knew what a trumpet looked like but had little idea about all those other intriguing shinny instruments.

A problem at the time was that the student had to provide his or her own instrument. I knew this would be a real burden to my mother who was alone after my father's death and had legal limits on her funds until we reached adult age. My father had left no will. However, my mother had insisted that education was foremost in our lives and that not to worry she would get an instrument. To make a long story short she was able to find a used Conn coronet (like a trumpet and approved by Mr. Mountain) for the price of 5 dollars. The bargain price was because the instrument had been dropped on a concrete floor by its previous owner smashing the bell of the horn. I hammered out the bell to where the damage did not interfere with the sound, at least the noise I put through it. However, big dents were very obvious to beholders. After metal polish and spit on the valves I got by. It was the instrument's heavy rectangular case of hardwood covered with leather that made my one mile walk home after school a burden.

The trumpet lesson was once a week from Mr. Mountain. Many years later I realized the ploy of my music teacher. He was preparing new recruits for his award-winning high school band. I'm not sure my hands or lips were really deciding factors, more so than the need to fill trumpet chairs in the high school band and orchestra. Nevertheless, I stuck with the trumpet and French horn through high school and college. While my young cousin Estes Felker excelled and was awarded the state championship as best trumpeter, I performed less well. I was not much better with the instrument than with those ball bats, golf clubs and sports stuff. Interestingly, Estes and I both gave up the trumpet when we entered medical school.

CHAPTER 5

Worth Street

An important time in my life, but oft forgotten, is the few years we lived on Worth Street in Cleveland. When my father and mother moved us "into town" in about 1936, we resided in three-fourths of a large, white clapboard Victorian house at 3315 Broad Street. The extra one-fourth of the house served as the Office and showroom of the funeral home. Come spring we packed up the car and moved back to the Home Place and Hughes Lake for the entire summer. When my father died in 1938, our mother was left to deal with the businesses, houses, farmland and timberland for which she had no experience or available help. In addition she was now a single mother with three small children ages 9, 6 and 3 years of age. Our father was never one to designate much of his work, so there was no one on hand who knew how to aid my mother.

Of major significance was that my father had left no will, thus requiring all property to be held in Probate Court until children reached 21 years of age. A key person, Judge Humphreys, sternly failed to help her with many of her problems and refused to allow any sale of property, except machinery, tools, vehicles, crops, etc. My mother turned to renting, something she could figure out and do on her own. She rented farmland to sharecroppers, who took advantage of her and provided a mere penance of income. She then rented out some rooms of the big house on Broad Street where we lived until she accrued enough money to buy a bargain house behind us on Worth Street. She would repair the dilapidated and abandoned place to a livable state, move us into it and rent the remainder of the big house.

At this time in Cleveland the main and best street was Ocoee St. that proceeded through the town from one end to the other. One block away and parallel to Ocoee was Broad Street. One block behind and parallel to Broad was the much smaller and less well-kept Worth Street. Near her new purchase was Pedro Elrod's Auto Repair Shop. Pee-Wee Engle's Food Store, a one room convenient store was located on Millie's property (about 2 acres which she purchased for about $1,500), so she became the proprietor of the building, a source for a little more rent. The house was a one-story square frame dwelling with a sagging front porch and overgrown with weeds and vines. The color was gray due to weathering of the wood that had never been painted. The place was called the Stoops house. The former owner, Mr. Stoops accidently killed himself while crawling under the house with a shotgun to kill rats. Somehow, eventually the do-it-yourself mother and children transformed the wreck into a clean white cottage with flowers in the yard.

A large vegetable garden was kept by my mother as a source of our food supply, with an occasional Nehi Orange, Royal Crown Cola or Coca Cola treat from Pee-Wee's ice box. She bought a cow and pastured it on the backside of the yard corralled with a barbed wire fence. I recall the dark night when she and I led the cow quietly through back streets of Cleveland from a farm three miles away to our house. I was a high school freshman very much in fear of being seen.

You may be surprised to learn that at no time in my life did I ever consider myself and my family as being poor or in poverty. None of us gave any thought of the FDR welfare "charity" in this post-depression era. We never ever considered ourselves to be candidates for welfare. We were just reasonably well-to-do people without much money. There were a lot of people like us. Though not easy, this widowed mother provided essentials for her children to live with dignity, attend college, including medical school for two, and enjoy long productive lives, without one cent from any government agency, without social security, without health insurance, and without a loan or mortgage of any kind. In fact, one hurdle for her was the governmental court system with an irresponsible judge who added to her burdens. Her financial philosophy was simply **"don't buy it until you can pay for it."**

While Worth Street was perhaps as far as the Hugheses ever got from beautiful Anglesey, Wales, some good times were found here. Neighborhood friends and playmates like Bitsy Million, Jack Elrod, Donald Haskell, Billy Gene White, and Glenn Franks had great times by just being together. Without much begging Millie often had kids to our house to spend the night on weekends. She was in the midst of us, telling her spellbinding ghost stories by fireside, providing eagerly consumed snacks of apples, pears or biscuit and sausage. Young people always liked her because she liked them.

We were allowed to listen together to a few radio programs including my favorites, The Lone Ranger, The Shadow, Charlie Chan, Amos and Andy and Fiber McGee and Mollie. I don't recall any news reports during this time. The boys had in common a passion for Comic Books, or "Funny Books" as some would say. Superheroes like Batman, Captain Marvel, Superman, Spider Man and Flash Gordon were favorites we traded back and forth, read and re-read. Second-line was Dick Tracy and the Green Hornet. Crisp new copies cost ten cents each. I'm still convinced a couple of my childhood buddies would never have learned to read were it not for comic books.

One literary level higher than the Comic Book was the "Big Little Book," a hardback book about two inches thick, but only about 4 by 5 inches in height and width. Each page was a cartoon with caption. I recall that our teacher's response to Jack Elrod's book report from a Big Little Book left no doubt as to future of his brilliant idea to save his buddies from those burdensome book reports.

Especially influential to boys in Cleveland was The Boy Scouts of America. Most boys participated, with weekly troop meetings at a local church and summer camping trips to lakes and trails of the Great Smoky Mountains. East Tennessee was ideal for scouting. The following powerful welcome to new Scouts by Ben H. Love, Chief Scout Executive, so accurately puts scouting into perspective that I quote it here.

"When you become a Boy Scout, something important happens to you. You aren't just joining an organization. You're entering a world full of exciting adventures. You belong to a group of friends that wants to go places and do things.

"As a Scout, you'll hike and camp, learn how to live in the out-of-doors, and discover many ways to care for the land. You can cook your meals over a camp stove and identify all kinds of plants and animals that are a part of our environment. No matter what happens, you'll know how to take care of yourself. You'll develop strength, confidence and good judgment. And, you can find out how it feels to be a leader.

"Scouting experiences will help you discover that you can make good things happen in your life by planning and setting goals and then reaching for them. You're in charge of yourself and your experiences, and there's no limit to what you can do – if you just put your mind to it."

I am typing the following statements from memory of what I learned some 75 years ago as a Boy Scout to illustrate the life-long impact these principles had on my life as well as other boys.

THE SCOUT OATH:

On my honor I will do my best
To do my duty to God and my country
And to obey the Scout Law;
To help other people at all times;
To keep myself physically strong,
Mentally awake, and morally straight.

THE SCOUT LAW:

A scout is trustworthy, loyal, helpful, friendly, courteous, kind, obedient, cheerful, thrifty, brave, clean and reverent.

THE SCOUT MOTTO: "Be Prepared!"

Especially enjoyable were the summer camping trips our Troop 77 took in the Great Smoky Mountains between Cleveland and Gatlinburg. The lakes were clear and cool. The one sport I always enjoyed was swimming in the mountains as well as Hughes Lake. I actually was a pretty good swimmer. While many camping and fishing stories come to mind, I'll mention only one because it reflects the important comradery of young boys who were the closest of friends.

As I recall there were some dozen or so boys undertaking a 10-day survival camp at Lake Chilhowee **(FIG. 5-A)** located high in the Smokies. Each Scout was required to plan and procure all supplies for the trip. Parents and others were not allowed to help the planning. The unchangeable rule was that we had to survive with what we brought. The motto of "Be Prepared" was the premise of the camp. We used an open shelter built of logs by the CCC corps of FDR. We each hung our hammocks in the shelter during the last day of the camp because of a slow persistent rain throughout the night. For the past two days our food supply had dwindled to cans of pork and beans. All the good stuff was gone and it was pork and beans for breakfast, lunch and dinner

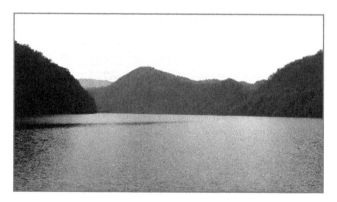

FIG. 5-A: Lake Chilhowee, TN – site of Troop 77 camping trip and famous contest (Courtesy Jim Negus, TWRA).

As we hung like bats in our hammocks suspended in the damp shelter and the hour was approaching midnight, conversations began to wane. Then, almost as a revival phenomenon, the physiological activities of the human gastrointestinal tract became activated in epidemic proportions. The first highly audible explosive flatus caused hilarious laughter. Soon events became competitive and Randall Hayes suggested we begin a "Farting Contest". The trooper who had the largest number of farts between now and 6:00 am would win.

"Win what?" the crowd asked.

"A Merit Badge!" suggested Randall. "We'll create new merit badge, The Farting* Merit Badge, for excellence in farting."

I don't recall the final winning number, but it was well above 25 farts and was won by my good friend Bobby Chestnut. Bobby's father was an important fireman in Cleveland and I often thought how proud he must have been of his son.

*NOTE: Perhaps most of you, except Greg, blush at the mention of this four-letter word. I apologize if you are offended, but you have no reason to be. Fart is a perfectly good word, one of the oldest in the English vocabulary with Indo-European origin (German, *furzen* or *ferzen*). It appears often in Geoffrey Chaucer's **Canterbury Tales** and Benjamin Franklin wrote an essay on the topic for the Royal Academy of Brussels in 1781, urging scientific study. It's like the other four-letter word for urine; both were considered proper even in scientific use before the latter part of the 19th century.

I would be remiss to deprive our grandchildren and subsequent generations of the saga of Joe's horse that occurred on the Worth Street premises. I preface the story by stating my intent is to point out the imaginative genius and fortitude of my little brother Joe (Hee! Hee!).

At around four years of age or so little Joe was heart-set on having a pony or a horse. He wanted his own pony and rode stick horses *in lieu* of the real thing. One fall day my uncle and mother's brother French Collett, who lived nearby came to the back door and said,

"Millie, take a look down in your cow pasture."

"Is that Joe?"

"Yes, he's been down there for half an hour or so."

"What's he doing?"

"He's digging a hole."

"What for?"

"To plant a horse."

"What do you mean?"

"I just went down to see what he was doing. He's very busy and excited. He found a dried stool excreted from a horse down the street. He collected it in your milk bucket and brought it home to plant in your cow pasture. He figured he could plant the horse stool and grow a horse. He brought it to your pasture so that when it grows up it can't run away."

Without saying much Joe went to the pasture daily until the weather turned cold. One winter day my mother secretly placed a small white porcelain horse statue she had bought at Woolworth's 5 & 10 Store, on the fecal burial site.

When the excited little boy led his mama to the pasture and pointed to the creation, she said something like, "Oh, Joe, you have a little horse, but it is frozen. You'll have to try again in the spring."

CHAPTER 6
Church and State

I was born a Methodist and a Republican, as were all Hugheses in Bradley County. We just considered it a birthright from John Wesley and Abraham Lincoln. The vast majority of us have held to these beliefs throughout life, with a rare backslider to the Presbyterians. Discussion of religion and politics rarely occurred in our family circles because we all agreed with each other. It was only after my mother's sister Clara married Darius Felker, a Democrat and a Baptist, that any reason to discuss politics arose. I point out that Darius was not a Hughes, but related through the Collett side of the family.

Nowadays, the politically correct and freethinking folk would consider me to have been deprived of the opportunity to choose for myself religious and political disciplines, rather than to just be "assigned" a role from birth. I have thought a lot about this and considered the options. Being of sound mind most of my life I believe I have had adequate opportunity for more than 80 years to make changes if I wished to do so. No one would stop me. I'm still satisfied and pleased that I was started off in the right direction.

I cannot recall going to church until we moved to Cleveland when I was about six years old. I expect I must have gone at least on occasion to the one-room wooden Sugar Creek Church near the Home Place, but I have no memory of it. While I think of my parents as dedicated Christians and church supporters, I can rarely recall them attending church, except perhaps for my mother in her senior years. Nevertheless, once in Cleveland she insisted that Katherine, Joe and I attend the First Methodist Church and sent us there on our own. Our house at 3315 Broad Street was ideally located for church going, probably due to careful planning by our parents. **(FIGS. 6-A to 6-C)**

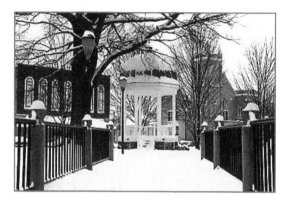

FIG. 6-A: Johnston Park between Broad and Ocoee Streets in Cleveland, as viewed in winter from our front porch on Broad Street. Notice the background buildings on Ocoee Street beginning on the right with the First Methodist Church, to the left of which is the top of the building housing the Princess Movie Theatre and at the end of the block is the Cherokee Hotel (not shown). Along the north side of the Park were a small grocery store and the Speck Hospital (not shown) where my father died. On the south side of the park was the home (not shown) of the kindly Judge Bean and family. His daughter, Leah, was my Spanish teacher in high school and his pretty granddaughters from Macon, GA visited in the summer and became life-long friends of Katherine, Joe and myself.

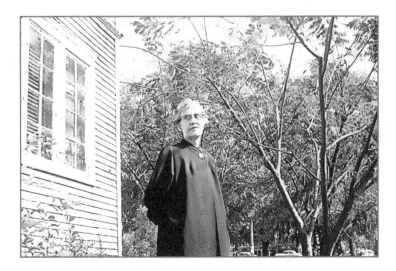

FIG. 6-B: Millie at age 70 years in front yard at Broad St. with Johnson Park in background.

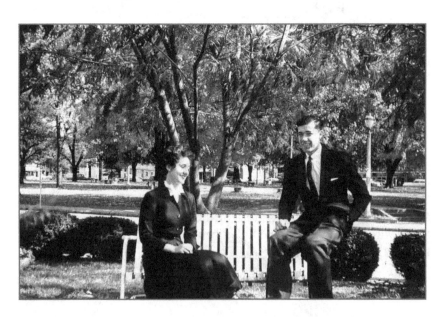

FIG. 6-C: My sister and brother, Katherine and Joe, at college age in front yard on Broad St.

The entire block in front of us between Broad Street and Ocoee Street had been donated by the Johnston Family to Cleveland as a City Park. It was intended as a place to walk and rest. From these pictures I can recall almost all of my life in Cleveland until I left for college in 1948. Sitting on the swing on our front porch my mother would regularly watch her children trek across the Park to church on Sunday and to the movie theater on Saturday afternoon (all afternoon). Candy bars could be bought at the food store (Cook's or Pee Wee's) before reaching the theater. The theater was filled with boys who watched the feature movie repeated two or three times during the afternoon. Most of my friends lived nearby and could convene by our secret whistle (a shrill "Pee-o-weet").

The First Methodist Church played an important role in my life and many people are not forgotten, even though I can't acknowledge them here. I'll mention three people I recall as especially influential.

Miss Alice White was a petite, soft-spoken lady a little older than my mother who was my first Sunday school teacher. I and my four or five classmates were probably between 7 and 8 years old and met for an hour before church service in a small dimly lit room in the basement of the church. To this day I can't identify a single attribute of Miss Alice that causes her to become so fixed in my memory that I name her here. She was not a dynamic person who entertained us, never brought treats to eat, we never played games, never told funny stories, we never sang the usual "Jesus Loves Me Songs," and she had never heard of the Lone Ranger and Roy Rogers. The hour was the same Sunday after Sunday. The classroom décor was devoid of educational items, with the exception some 4 or 5 colorful storybooks and a *Holy Bible,* which Miss Alice brought, and spread before us on the low level round table around which we sat. All the books were beautifully illustrated stories of Jesus. I can only remember that she read and talked about Jesus in a way that caused us to listen and come to love Miss Alice.

Rev. Elton Jones was a young handsome and charismatic minister who brought a new spirit of dedication and enthusiasm to the church. I recall his role among the youth who flocked to his services and that caused me to become, because of choice, more and more involved in the church. The Methodist Youth Fellowship every Sunday night and choir practice every Wednesday night after Prayer Meeting were added to activities I wanted to do. The choir moved me to a bass voice and taught me how to enunciate and speak to minimize my strong East Tennessee accent, but I fell short of excellence in vocal performance.

I now realize that Rev. Elton Jones not only appealed to the youth but to the elderly as well. In fact, my mother began to attend the Sunday morning sermons, and I know he often praised her for her role as a mother. I now believe we were fond of him because he sincerely was fond of us. I think there must be something basic to human behavior in the *quid pro quo* concept. Many years later after Rev. Elton Jones had moved on to more prestigious pulpits and then retired, he gladly travelled a long distance back to Bradley County to conduct the funeral service of our mother, and her burial at rural Sugar Creek Cemetery.

Rev. Ralph Johnson was a visiting evangelist who came to First Methodist Church for a week of evening revival services. In addition to compelling sermons he had a dynamic operatic baritone voice and had sung in important concerts. When he sang "The Holy City" the windows shook. He never knew me but I attended all the services. It was during this week that, at age 13 years, I decided to live my life as a Christian. The decision was within my mind as I sat still in the pew. I didn't stand to be recognized or go down to an altar, but the decision was firm. From that time on I controlled outbreaks of temper I sometimes experienced, developed some degree of compassion for those around me and adopted the Beatitudes as guidelines for life. Later, I often wondered why I had not had the powerful emotional experience others experienced in "being saved". I have come to the conclusion that the magnitude of such an experience is related directly to the extent of "sins" one has committed. Maybe my life was dull (I don't think so), but I could not recall any big time sins. I was always honest, never stole anything, not an alcoholic or on drugs, never killed anybody or committed adultery, and was never in jail. Furthermore, I was a Bradley County Hughes born a Methodist and a Republican. So, I had no big tears to move me down front to an altar. I believe God understands this.

I include in this chapter some comments on the State, meaning Government, because of the striking differences in Church and State now and the time of my youth. I'll mention some aspects of governmental impact on my life in these early days and let you the devoted readers make comparison to present-day circumstances. I believe my knowledge and understanding as a teenager, of the United States government and world affairs was greater than that of some of the later generations.

I go back to my world around Johnston Park in Cleveland to comment further on another important institution in my youth. I may sound sacrilegious, but I'll say anyway that The Princess Movie Theater was close to the Church in affecting the evolution of my life. It was here I spent almost all of my Saturday afternoons. Routinely, I spent Saturday morning collecting from the customers on my paper route. Then, at least two buddies and I would pay 10 cents each for admission to The Princess Movie Theater. The Saturday movies were always westerns (Roy Rogers, Hopalong Cassidy, Gene Autry, The Lone Ranger, etc.) where good and evil were clearly delineated and good always won. Of importance I realize now, but not then, was a ten-minute **"Newsreel"** run after each movie.

The **Newsreel** showed world events of the **past week.** We all <u>had</u> to watch the news if we were to see the movie. My smart history teacher, Miss Rogers, gave grade credit to boys who turned in a paragraph summary of the week's news.

I was eleven years old on December 7, 1941 when the Japanese attacked Pearl Harbor, enhancing World War II. I saw **weekly** reports of **all** of World War II vividly reported at The Princess Theater. We saw the battles, the bombing and the devastation directly on film by reporters, like Ernie Pyle, and many others who brought the unspun facts without political distortion to us the people. Truth, accuracy and honesty were hallmarks of our news journalists of the day, perhaps a factor half a century later in Tom Brokaw's designation of us as "The Greatest Generation," of all time.

Four years of my life in Cleveland (1941-1945) were profoundly influenced by "The State", that is the federal government, due to World War II. Current-day issues of civil rights, patriotism, law and order, immigration, loyalty and service to country, right and wrong, lines between Church and State, and political correctness seem totally foreign to our circumstances in the 1940s.

The War caused our town to become depleted of young men who were drafted into military services. This resulted in shortages of store clerks, doctors, teachers, policemen, firemen, grocers, farmers, mill workers and others. Younger people and older people tended to fill the spaces. National shortages of resources became evident and citizens were asked to sacrifice for our country. Rationing was imposed by law. Government stamps were issued monthly to each citizen for limited supplies of food and gasoline. Luxuries were just not available – no candy bars, ice cream, no nylon hose, etc. A Hersey's chocolate bar was something to die for. Milk became known as "blue john" because dilution with water took away the whiteness. New clothing was no longer thought about. I recall in my new weekend job as a clerk at Millers' Department store, Men's Department; we received a small supply of shirts from the Wings Shirt Co. with a new 'Duke of Windsor' collar, designed for the war effort. By removing 2 to 3 inches off the tips of pointed collars, more cotton material was made available to our men in service. To this day I wear shirts with the widespread collar that evolved from the war.

Even Cleveland became worried about possible air invasion by Germans, Japanese, or both. The Federal Government established an active Civil Defense Program in Bradley County, as well as all U.S counties. Bomb shelters were established, practices for blackouts and air raid events were regularly undertaken. Our Boy Scout Troop 77 was active in drives to collect scrap paper and tinfoil needed by the government for some new "re-cycling" procedures under development.

My buddies and I really got into the war effort. We learned to recognize silhouettes of all foreign aircraft as well as U. S fighters and every boy had a pair of binoculars. We collected enough newspapers and tin foil to fill our garage almost to the ceiling and wall-to-wall. Shortages of tin and paper led to recycling efforts. How relieved my mother was when an army truck came to empty the wood garage of the potential fire hazard! Members of our Boy Scout Troop 77 each received the Dwight D. Eisenhower Medal for our contribution to the war effort.

As might be expected, many people in our area thought it was a big over-kill to focus on foreign invasion. After all, why would Germany, Italy and Japan have any interest at all in our little town in the southeast corner of Tennessee? Several citizens spoke out about City funds being spent on protecting our city against foreign invaders.

"No Jap or German ever heard of Cleveland, Tennessee," a citizen said at a town meeting. "Mr. Mayor, if you must do something, I suggest you put a canon in the city park, so we can shoot the enemy when he invades." The audience laughed.

Little did they know! Little did I know! Little did anyone know of the absolutely earth-shaking events beginning to evolve some 80 miles up the highway from Cleveland? It was here the most profound anti-war strategy of any leader or of any government in the history of the world was evolving. Soon after the Pearl Harbor attack, President Franklin Delano Roosevelt got the U.S. Congress to secretly fund the development of a new weapon with the potential to end World War II and hopefully future wars. The effort required massive and rapid expansion of scientific, research and military resources, including the secret acquisition of 60,000 acres of land in the foothills of the Appalachian Mountains of East Tennessee, just north of Cleveland.

By one means or another land was acquired from citizens by the government and cleared. New structures were built and tens of thousands of people from all over the world were brought to the East Tennessee site. Secrecy was the foremost rule of the day. The entire area, not included on maps and unnamed except for the "Clinton Engineering Works" was enclosed by a high-level gated security wall, patrolled by soldiers and required governmental clearance for entry. It seemed everything about it was a clandestine operation. No news reporters were allowed on the premises. However, one reporter-photographer Ed Wescott was authorized to become a permanent inside resident to record the historical events.

Most employees of three rapidly built manufacturing plants (X-10, Y-12, and K-25) were not aware of the goal of the overall project or how their specific jobs contributed to it. While they knew they were working on a secret war effort project for the U. S. government, few of them had ever heard of Uranium and an Atomic Bomb was something in science fiction. The major labor-intensive push to separate Uranium 235, needed for a bomb, from Uranium 238 was ceaseless 24 hours a day and 7 days-a-week and basic to the Manhattan Project. By 1945, some 75,000 people now lived and worked at the site, soon to be revealed on maps as **OAK RIDGE, TENNESSEE.** They saw hundreds of rail cars filled with ore enter the plants, but saw nothing leave because the important component amounted to fleck in a bottle.

In July, 1945 the accumulated small precious amounts of Uranium 235 were taken from **OAK RIDGE, TENNESSEE** to **LOS ALAMOS, NEW MEXICO**, and placed in a nuclear bomb dubbed "Little Boy."

On August 6, 1945 we sat spellbound by our radios listening to the announcement that the United States had dropped an Atomic Bomb on Hiroshima, Japan, destroying the city. Three days later a second bomb was dropped on Nagasaki, Japan that led within a few days to the surrender of Japan, ending World War II. Local political cartoonists depicted the "Little Boy" bomb with a highly visible boiler mark reading, "**Made in Oak Ridge, Tennessee, USA.**"

Much more can be said about these critical war years in Cleveland with interesting stories about our family, but I don't have time to say it now – after all, I'm 84 years old, you know, and I need to get to chapter 7.

CHAPTER 7

High School and College Years: 1944-1954

To continue my saga in chronological order, I am now up to about 14 years of age (1944-45), graduated from the 8th grade at Arnold Memorial School and starting in the 9th grade at Bradley Central High School **(FIG. 7-A)** on N. Ocoee Street, about two miles from our home on Broad Street.

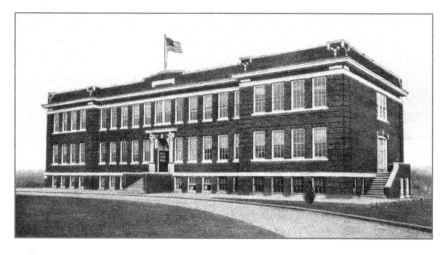

FIG. 7-A: Bradley Central High School, N. Ocoee St., Cleveland, Tennessee (*OCOEEAN YEARBOOK*).

Surely, you say, his year in high school will be better than what we've been reading. This will be where the good stuff begins. A car, driver's license, dating, pep rallies, hayrides, proms, football games, homecomings, clusters of friends, parties, popularity, etc. Well, indeed my four years of high school were memorable, and I am grateful to all those excellent teachers and fellow students who contributed to my welfare. However, as I try to write about it I find it very difficult.

I got out my old **OCOEEAN YEARBOOK,** orange and black "Bradley Bear" trivia and a few photos of old friends and pondered how to start. I thought to myself, "I can cover all this in one paragraph." I passed each grade, made the National Honor Society but was never a truly outstanding student of valedictorian status. The 1948 **OCOEEAN YEARBOOK** credits show I was a member and officer of the Bradley High School Band, lettered in Band, was President of the Spanish Club, Vice-president of the Dramatics Club and member of the Glee Club, Aeronautics Club, Music Club and Pep Club (everyone was a member of the Pep Club). The very popular and pretty Sarah Park and geekish I were dubbed "Most Dignified" couple, which says a lot about my high school lifestyle. Overall, considering high school activities of the day, among the 130 graduating seniors I would consider myself to be among the fortunate average. College years were similarly mundane. So what else can I say?

When I mentioned to Carla that I was having trouble in writing about high school and college years and that I was coming to realize these were maybe the least enjoyable years of my life, she said with her usual wisdom, like her mother, **"Well, just say so!!** Someday it might encourage a grandchild or great-grandchild to know this." So, that's what I'm going to do.

The high school freshman year (1944-45) was associated with important changes in my life. It was a change from my little world around Johnston Park, Broad, Ocoee and Worth Streets to the "distant" suburb of North Cleveland, two miles away and accessible to me only by foot at the time. Moreover, I was entering a somewhat different social culture, the first of many more to come.

I found the proper Bradley High freshman didn't spend his Saturday afternoons watching Hopalong Cassidy and Roy Rogers. Comic books were uncouth. Only an occasional feature movie shown during the week at The Princess Theater (not the Bohemia Theater down the street) was politically posh. However, these "week-day" movies were remarkable and elevated my cultural status a peg or so. How fortunate I was to have benefited from the movie production era of the 1940s.

I began to read hardback books from the library, phase out comics, and to choose a movie because of the cast of actors as much as the plot – Humphrey Bogart, Lionel Barrymore, Sidney Greenstreet, Orson Wells, James Stewart, Spencer Tracy, Katherine Hepburn, and Henry Fonda, to mention a few. However, weeknight prices were high – 20 cents per person and candy was not allowed and I no longer had my paper route. The epic **Gone with the Wind** cost a record-breaking 35 cents. My old neighborhood buddies were not particularly interested in the non-Saturday movies. I was able to only occasionally attend such a movie.

World War II ended in 1945 and the fascination of civil defense, searching for German spies and watching the weekly **Newsreels** faded. I moved out of the Boy Scouts because of age.

Now, Joe, Katherine and I would be going to different schools. Some of my buddies were assigned to a school in south Cleveland and I would likely see little of them in the future. Bradley Central High was considered rather large at the time **(FIG. 7-A)**, maybe about 600 students (currently over 1,600 students). While most of my Arnold Memorial School classmates for eight years entered the Bradley High freshman class, they were diluted out with incoming students from more than five other elementary schools throughout the county. So, in a sense, my social life had to be re-created, though this was not a conscious plan by any means.

Serendipitously, Mr. Mountain's pro *bono* trips to Arnold and my five-dollar, beat-up coronet, determined the direction of my life through high school. Unfortunately, Mr. Mountain died before I reached high school. The War had taken most of the male teachers by military draft, so tryouts for the Bradley High School Band were held by three female teachers, not primarily involved in the music program. I expect these circumstances were key factors in my being accepted into the trumpet section of the band. It was rumored that one of these dear ladies had left her hearing aid at home on the try-out day.

I'm convinced that it was not just music that brought together some five young men in 1945 who would become very close friends throughout the next half decade or so. Foremost among these was Crill Higgins, perhaps the closest friend of my life. Others were Eddy Nicholson (trumpet), James Albert ("Dee") Watenbarger (trombone) and Max Weaver (drums). Somehow, we ended up as the five officers of the high school band **(FIG.7-B)**.

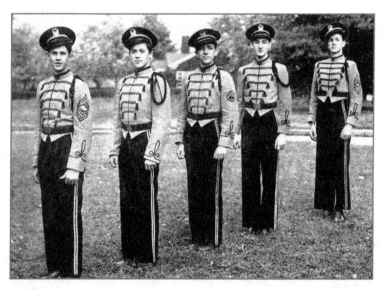

FIG. 7-B: Officers of the Bradley Central High School Band, 1947 – L to R = Max Cooper, James Albert Watenbarger, Crill Higgins, Walter Hughes and Eddy Nicholson (*OCOEEAN YEARBOOK, 1947).*

Crill Higgins had not attended Arnold Memorial School, but I came to know him because his parents, Harley and Sarah Higgins and my mother had been friends for several years. In fact, in their youth, his father and my mother had dated for a brief time.

Crill was the most "natural" musician among us. His main instrument was the piano because it allowed him to perform exciting music as well as compose and arrange, but he also mastered the clarinet and several other instruments during high school. I cannot recall a moment when Crill seriously considered any role in life that did not have music as his profession. At the same time, I never recall any obvious ambition to become a celebrity. All he seemed to want was to be constantly involved in music. He was handsome with a delightful personality and great sense of humor. During our high school years we became bound like brothers and were almost inseparable friends. We registered for the same classes, had lunch together, attended the same events together, and at times wore identical clothing.

In those days we tended to go out in groups of boys and girls, rather than "dating" in pairs. Crill and I tended to hang with the music crowd. By the time of our senior year nature had taken its course and Crill had fallen deeply and permanently in love with one of our buddies, Joyce Ellis. Even in high school Joyce, a beautiful and lovable blond, stood above all others as a concert-grade pianist. She commanded the stage alone.

All of my high school buddies went into musical fields except for me. I expect none of them loved music any more than I, but I just lacked any desire to become a performer or teacher of music. That is fortunate because I lacked the natural talent of Crill and the others and was left to the plight of the untalented ending up as scientists, engineers, doctors, lawyers, etc.

My college major and profession choice came after long soul searching, researching and repeated pro and con lists. My short list included Architecture, Journalism, Clergy and Medicine. If I chose what I "would really like to do" all day it would probably have been Architecture. I was always fascinated with buildings. This was enhanced every day during my walk to high school for four years.

FIGURES 7-C to 7-I (FROM PHOTOSOFCLEVELAND.COM, CREATED BY PHIL LEA) show some buildings I walked passed twice-daily going to and from school. Cleveland was unique among small southern towns of the time in having high quality in art, music and architecture. I chose Medicine because it offered altruistic opportunities.

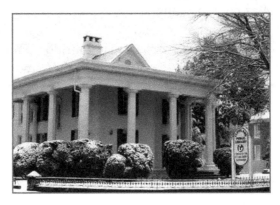

FIG. 7-C: On my walk to high school - Cleveland Library

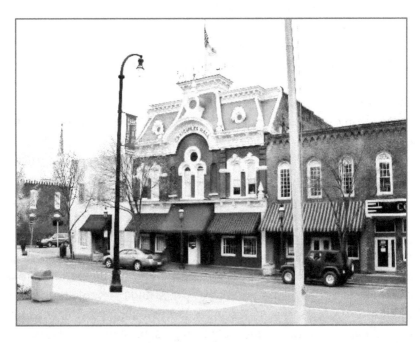

FIG. 7-D: On my walk to high school - Craigmiles Hall (Original Opera House 1878).

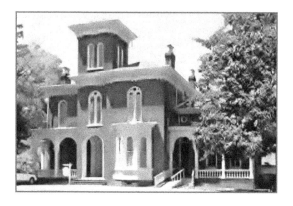

FIG. 7-E: On my walk to high school – the Craigmiles House

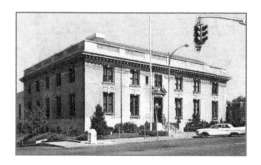

FIG. 7-F: On my walk to high school: Cleveland Post Office, Broad St.

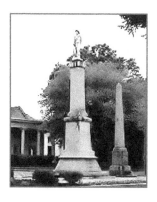

FIG. 7-G: On my walk to school; Confederate Monument, junction Broad St. and Ocoee St.

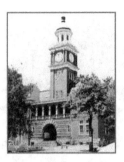

FIG. 7-H: On my walk to high school: Bradley County Court House, Broad St.

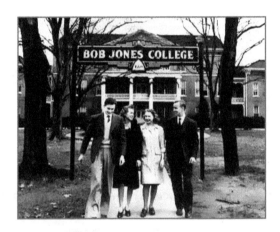

FIG. 7-I: On my walk high to school – Bob Jones College (Now Lee University).

After graduation four of us headed for the same college, Tennessee Polytechnic Institute ("Tennessee Tech") in Cookeville, TN., three as music majors and me a pre-med major. This state college was a favorite conduit for Bradley High students and had a good reputation for success of its graduates. Indeed, all my friends had successful careers in music and I made it to medical school.

After college Crill and Joyce married and returned to Cleveland where they contributed their remarkable talents for the rest of their lives. Crill became an icon for almost half a century as

Music and Band Director of the High Schools and surrounding school systems in southeast Tennessee and northeast Georgia. His award-winning bands performed often nationally including half-time shows at the Orange Bowl and at the U.S. Bicentennial Celebration in Washington, DC. His approach to music was much more than hitting the right note at the right time. He prepared the way for beautiful music and took charge of progress, often introducing himself at fund-raisers saying, "My name is Crill Higgins and I teach enthusiasm!" **(FIG. 7-J.)**

During my first two years of college at Tennessee Tech I was able to accrue enough credits to qualify early for medical school, so I applied and was accepted to start in 1950. I had a part-time job in the Library, played in the Tech Band and was awarded the 1950 Gold Medal in Biology for academic excellence. The content of this sentence seems to be my total recall of the college because my life was spent between the dorm and classroom.

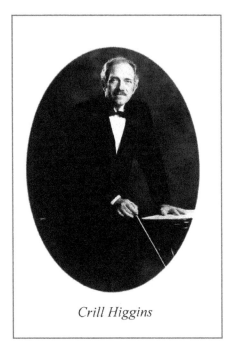

Crill Higgins

FIG. 7-J: Crill Higgins

The year 1950 was another turning point in my life and a major one. Sadly, I had an almost complete severance from all of my close friends of the past and music. I never saw them again, except for Crill and Joyce on very rare occasions, due to wide geographic distances and the disparity of our professions. I sold my trumpet and I lost track of movies until the evolution of television years later.

Now I was moving to a much larger school and city. The University Of Tennessee College Of Medicine was one of the largest medical schools in the U.S. at the time. It was located in the city of Memphis, more than 300 miles from Cleveland and in humid flatland of West Tennessee on the Mississippi River, strikingly different from my beloved Wales-like mountainous East Tennessee. Also, the music in Memphis was different from mine – something of a vulgar noise called blues and jazz.

Of the nearly one million people in the metropolitan Memphis area, I knew one of them, Vernon "Pete" Bryant. He came with me from Tennessee Tech and had been a football star at Bradley High School. Pete was entering Dental School and we became roommates for a year in the notorious Manassas Dormitory facing Nathan Bedford Forrest Park on Manassas St. The signs reading "Pending Condemnation" posted around the dorm were bothersome. An explanation was that the area had been condemned but funds were not yet available to remove it. Pete was a very good friend and later was a prominent dentist in Cleveland, TN for the rest of his life. I'm now beginning to realize that almost everyone who moved away from Cleveland eventually came back.

The first statement in the Dean's Welcome to our class at Medical School suggested each of us look to the person on the right and then to the person sitting on the left and to become aware that one of the three would not be graduating with the class. This line, probably gleaned from an army boot camp, was not one any of us wrote home about, and did little to instill confidence in fairness of the educational system. Nevertheless, the die was cast and the four-year race was on with every student totally dedicated to pass examinations, make good grades, achieve faculty approval at any cost, obey instructions, stay out of trouble and survive by passing grades quarter by quarter.

In 1950 few of the buildings were equipped with air conditioning. Large fans circulated the formaldehyde-laden air of the cadaver dissection laboratories where we worked in groups of four per specimen. Organic chemistry laboratories lacked chemical exhaust hoods during the urea cycle experiments. In my second year I moved to the large one room "attic suite" (without air-conditioning) of the Alpha Kappa Kappa Fraternity House on Adams Ave. shared with my classmates Paul Estes and Harold Vann who were true scholars and regularly ranked first and second in class grades. Our lives were spent almost totally in class or attic room.

In my senior year I was fortunate to get a heavily sought-after job as an extern at the prestigious Campbell's Clinic for Orthopedics, a world leader in this field. The job provided free room and board, but no salary. I was on duty every third night as an x-ray technician, to shave and prep surgery sites and assist the surgeon as needed.

By pursing the continuous quarter system through summers I was able to finish medical school in three and a half years causing me to receive my M.D. degree in March 1954, just shortly before my 24th birthday on May 16, 1954. However, this created a problem. My general rotating internship at the Knoxville General Hospital, back in my beloved East Tennessee, at the home campus of the University of Tennessee, 60 miles from Cleveland, 20 miles from Oak Ridge and perched in the beautiful Smoky Mountains did not begin until July 1, 1954. While a three-month vacation at home would have been heavenly, my finances would cover no more than two or three days of such luxury, so I took a four-month locum *tenems* job with two senior general practice physicians in Tazewell, W. Virginia.

The four-month experience in the hills of West Virginia and Virginia was remarkably valuable to me. The excellent clinical training at the University of Tennessee prepared students to take care of sick patients, more so, than in theoretical concepts and research. So, as a licensed physician I was able to do general practice with

Drs. Rufus Britton and Mary Elizabeth Johnson in Tazwell. Many times I was alone with very sick people and there was no one, literally no one, to treat them except myself. I delivered babies at home and in our office clinic. Overall, I recalled having delivered more than 100 babies during my pre-academic life.

One of my most memorable experiences at Tazewell began one Saturday when I was called to the local jail to see a drunken inmate who had slashed his wrist in a suicidal attempt. His wrist was limp and tendons were dangling loose. I controlled the bleeding, cleaned and dressed the wound, splinted the wrist, gave a tetanus shot and called the Emergency Room at the nearest hospital with a surgeon in Bluefield, West VA, informing them I was sending the patient for urgent treatment. This was at about 4:00 pm. At about 11:30 pm I received a call from the sheriff's office saying the surgeon in Bluefield had found the man uncontrollable and unwilling to receive treatment, so he sent him back to me. My practice colleagues were out of town. What to do? Time was becoming important because without proper surgical correction and closure infection would soon occur, likely leading to gangrene and possibly septic death. Unless I did something, nothing would be done.

From a footlocker in my room of "stuff" I brought with me to Tazewell (all of my worldly possessions) I found a Ciba Symposium publication on the anatomy of the hand and wrist, magnificently illustrated by the famous medical artist, Frank Netter. Also, I was pleased to find an old portable music stand left from days of horn practice. With the aid of a guard from the jail, a lot of sedation and novacaine, Netter's drawings displayed on my music stand setting alongside me and the patient restrained on an exam table, I spent most of the night pulling retracted tendons from the forearm, trying to match with severed ends in the wrist and suture them together. Somehow, maybe by God's will, the patient survived. When I left at the end of June, he could move all fingers, except the small finger that had a contracture.

It wasn't until I completed the pressurized, examination-fixed, score-focused medical college system that I began to study and learn in a meaningful way. When I could choose what I wished to study and how I wished to study it I began to really learn medicine. From the writing of notes from medical journal articles on 3" x 5" index cards in the 1950s, to the advent of Xerox photocopies, and now the all- magnificent internet learning has become a precious opportunity for me.

CHAPTER 8

Internship and Residency (1954-1957)

Surely, you say, this is where some really good stuff will begin. We know all about interns and residents from television shows and movies – pretty nurses, love affairs, ambulance sirens, red alert emergencies, CPRs, pages from a loudspeaker, people saying "stat" a lot and doctors getting big hugs for saving lives. Well folks, you know I'm 84 years old, so I just can't remember some things about my internship 60 years ago. In those days, we interns were all un-married men living in quarters in the top floor of the hospital, wore hospital scrubs night and day, dined for free in the cafeteria and had access to a large pool table in the hall outside our quarters. I was on call six days a week plus every third night.

At the end of my internship in 1955 the old Knoxville General Hospital closed its doors, moved across town and changed its name (to The University of Tennessee Memorial Hospital). I assure you it was not because of something I did or didn't do, but I cherish the privilege of that historic year in Knoxville.

My internship was at the end of an era in another way. The tra-ditional year of training following medical school graduation had been the "rotating" internship, wherein the intern spent practice time rotating through departments of surgery, internal medicine, obstetrics, pediatrics, ear, nose and throat, etc. By the mid-1950s changes were coming about to introduce "straight" internships in which the intern spent the entire year in one specialty. The advantage was that those planning to specialize could be better prepared for a residency. The disadvantage was that the doctor would not be able to develop fully some basic general skills of clinical practice, such as surgery. I chose the rotating internship.

As specialists in medicine flourished so did the straight internship and the rotating programs diminished. Even though I went on to specialize in Pediatrics I never regretted my rotating internship during which I delivered several babies, did three or four appendectomies, pinned a fractured hip and learned many practical skills. Afterwards I felt greater confidence in providing broader care for children than with the more narrow experience.

Interestingly, social issues in medicine developing over the years limited to some extent the use of skills for which I was adequately trained. Malpractice suits were arising and doctors were becoming more cautious. A memorable anecdote from my rotating internship was a forecast of future issues. On the last day of the month during my Pediatrics rotation I admitted a young boy with acute otitis media and a bulging eardrum because of pus in the middle ear. I was preparing to do a simple myringotomy (incise the ear drum to let pus drain out), which I had been trained to do, and had done many times before. However, my attending staff doctor suggested I obtain an ENT consultant to do the procedure. I submitted the request to ENT department as per policy. The next morning I started my rotation on the ENT service, where I was handed the consultation request I had submitted several hours earlier. The ENT resident told me to answer the consult because he had never done a myringotomy in a child and I had. I did the procedure and the child recovered. I used this true story during my academic years to remind medical students to look realistically at what they are doing and to assure themselves that the consultant to whom they refer patients can do better than they.

The great pleasure of my time in Knoxville was its proximity to

Cleveland where I could visit my mother and sister Katherine. My brother Joe was now in Medical School in Memphis and they were living there alone. Katherine had also lived in Knoxville earlier as a student at the University of Tennessee, but decided to return home and stay with our mother.

I became interested in Pediatrics in Medical School because of influential faculty including, Drs. James N. Ettledorf, Thomas Mitchell and James G. Hughes. In the 1950s Ettledorf brought a scientific base to Memphis Pediatrics, demonstrating the impact of fluid and electrolyte infusion therapy and biochemical monitoring in reducing drastically the mortality from infantile diarrhea and dehydration during summer epidemics in Memphis infants. The remarkable results lay before us on the wards to observe. His research on renal diseases was innovative. Ettledorf was totally dedicated to medicine and teaching. He was loved, feared, admired, respected and demanded perfection from those around him. For decades to come he would command a favorite professor status from his students and colleagues who established **The James N. Ettledorf Award** in his honor and to bring outstanding visiting scientist-physicians to Memphis for lectures. This event continues as a highlight of the academic year where "Dr. E" is remembered.

"Dr. Tom" Mitchell was the most senior Pediatrician in Memphis and had served as Chairman of the Department of Pediatrics in years past. A slightly chubby, baby-faced, balding, man with keen and gleaming eyes, a vest decorated with a modest gold watch chain, and wearing meticulously clean rimless spectacles perched on the bridge of his nose and anchored from one side by a fine chain to his lapel, he toddled down the halls often with a few kids following. His lectures on the premature infant were given each quarter to students. I was privileged to attend and with others was mesmerized as he brilliantly and humbly talked about these "little bitty" babies, while holding a baby and demonstrating responses.

Dr. James G. Hughes, Chairman of the Department for many years was nationally and internationally renowned. He served as President of the American Academy of Pediatrics and made many contributions to the development of Pediatrics in Central and South America. He was a General in the U.S. Amy after World War II and his Pediatric Department was kept in good order. As far as I know he and I were not directly related, except possibly for some unknown Welsh bloodline common to all Hugheses.

At the time I began my residency in Pediatrics in 1955, training in Pediatrics at The University of Tennessee College of Medicine had been focused entirely at the Frank T. Tobey Children's Hospital, a large wing of the City-County John Gaston Hospital. However, in 1952 the long-sought new freestanding Le Bonheur Children's Hospital became available for approved residency training of UT residents in Pediatrics. I was accepted to the Le Bonheur arm along with two other new residents. For a period of time one Chief Resident was appointed to the larger Tobey program and another to the Le Bonheur program. When I became Chief at the Le Bonheur site in 1956-7, I received the lucrative stipend of $25 per month, plus nicer room and better food than my more prestigious counterpart at Tobey. Several years later the memorable Tobey was closed and Le Bonheur became the sole site for Pediatric training at UT.

With a promise that I'll tell you later about a fabulous love affair during my last year at Le Bonheur, I'd like to tell you now about a truly remarkable serendipitous event that actually determined my future career and lead me to the field of Infectious Diseases and academic medicine.

In the fall of 1956 I admitted a teenage African-American girl complaining of fever, sore throat and earache. The tonsils were red, swollen and covered with a grayish-white exudative membrane. The lymph nodes of the neck were enlarged and tender. These findings were typical of streptococcal tonsillitis, so treatment with penicillin was begun. Because she did not promptly respond as expected another diagnosis was considered. Diphtheria was excluded because of immunization and infectious mononucleosis because of negative blood tests. An evening searching the journals for rare causes of exudative tonsillitis yielded a list of tests that I ordered. Before the results were available I talked again to the patient and found that she had dressed rabbits for food a few weeks earlier. The entire illness was totally compatible with the diagnosis of **Tularemia, ("Rabbit Fever")** caused by the bacterium, *Francisella tularensis*, highly contagious from rabbit to man. Blood tests showed rising antibody titers to 1:320, then to 1:640 confirming the diagnosis. Treatment with terramycin resulted in a prompt response and cure.

Dr. Ettledorf was my Attending Staff and when I presented my case on bedside rounds and gave the unusual diagnosis of oropharyngeal tularemia, he broke out his happy smile and started staccato questions galore. Something outside the usual made his day. Of course I had read up on the case before rounds and was able struggle through the questions and discussion.

In the midst of rounds Dr. E said loudly, "Hughes, you need to write this case up for a medical journal – go through all the hospital records and analyze all the Memphis cases."

Ettledorf's directive startled me at first but then I became excited. Could I, the Bradley County farm boy, actually write and have published an article for a national medical journal? Dr. E didn't stop with a flippant suggestion. When I expressed my keen interest, he set up writing and review schedules with the ground rule that I, not he, would do all the writing. My first draft glowed red after his red crayon marker. I sat beside him while he went over every single mark telling me why it was there. The article entitled "Oropharyngeal Tularemia", by Walter T. Hughes and James N. Ettledorf, was published in the *Journal of Pediatrics* in 1957. During my residency I published two more articles with Dr. E's help and encouragement aiming me toward a career in academic medicine. Some four decades after I sat beside him as a resident I had the heart-warming honor of receiving the **1994 James N. Ettledorf Award** from the University of Tennessee College of Medicine.

Enter now serendipity. I had come close to a decision to subspecialize in Hematology. I realized that to succeed in academic medicine I must subspecialize. However, in late 1956 I was drafted into the U.S. Navy and would have to interrupt my residency. Dr. (General) James Hughes suggested I quickly volunteer to join the

U.S. Army where I would be allowed to complete my residency. I did.

On July 1, 1957 I became a Captain in the U.S. Army Medical Corps and was sent to Fort Sam Houston, in San Antonio, TX for basic training, learning how to march, shoot guns, crawl under barbed wire below machine gun fire, etc. At the end of the summer in Texas we were assigned to permanent posts for the next two years. Our troops were still in Korea and most inductees expected to be sent there. I was single and felt sure I would be on the boat to Korea.

Surprisingly, my assignment was to the Walter Reed Army Medical Unit at Ft. Detrick, MD, just 60 miles outside Washington, DC. This was the U.S. Government's top-secret Biological Warfare Research Laboratory. I could not begin duty until I had gone through top-secret clearance by FBI, etc. My first thought was that some mistake had occurred. I had become accustomed to having name confusion with Dr. James Hughes in Memphis. However, with time the rationale for the assignment became clear.

It seems *Francisella tularensis* was one of the most nearly ideal bacterial warfare agents. Other agents included *Bacillus anthracis* the cause of anthrax. All countries were aware of this. During this era of the "Cold War" with Russia the U.S. War Department learned that the Russians had a tularemia vaccine and were immunizing thousands of their population. They feared Russia might be preparing to attack the U. S. with *F. tularensis*. So, a research unit was being established at Ft. Detrick via the Walter Reed Institute of Research to develop and test a vaccine for the prevention of tularemia. Thus, when the word **tularemia** appeared on my resume my lot fell to the research team. The ensuing two years working with world greats in Microbiology and Infectious Diseases, committed me to a future in this field. So, I have never doubted that when Dr. E in Memphis said, "Hughes, you should write up this case!" my lot was cast.

Much more will be said about Ft. Detrick and tularemia later, but I must now get to the "good stuff" I promised.

CHAPTER 9

Jeanette

How can I tell you about a great love story when my words are clinical and don't fit the intended meaning? Poets have beautiful words but with meaningless definitions. They speak of broken and crying hearts; I speak of hearts that pump and beat. Among languages love is a unique word that is totalistic and all inclusive of its meaning and requires no modifiers. It is experienced by all, whether literate or illiterate. I can't define it, describe it or even understand it, but that's not necessary because love is to be experienced, one with another, not dissected and analyzed. More than anything now, I want to tell you of my love for my dear Jeanette, but words are lacking and you'll have to judge it from our lives together.

One Sunday morning in the spring of 1956 I decided to go to church. It was a beautiful day and I had not been outside Le Bonheur Children's Hospital in more than two weeks. I both worked and lived there. I had the whole day off and walked casually past the Victorian mansions on Adams Ave. to the historic First Methodist Church **(FIG. 9-A)** at the corner of Poplar and Second. It must have been March because Jonquils were in bloom and the air was fresh. I had not been to church much during the last two years and it felt good to be doing so now. I wore a dark brown blazer, tan gabardine pants, white dress shirt and yellow tie – not that I recall this but I know that was the only "Sunday" suit I owned at the time.

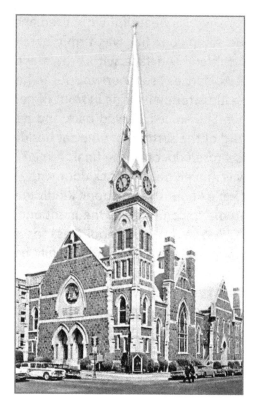

FIG. 9-A: First Methodist Church, Memphis.

I entered the back doors of the church just before the service started and found a seat on the back row and on the right side. The sloping floor to the pulpit allowed good visibility of the congregation. All women, young and old wore stylish colorful hats, matching gloves and fashionable dresses.

Standing for the first hymn, I was attracted to three young women about mid-way down on the left side of the sanctuary. More correctly, I was attracted to **one** of three young women. I was 26 years old, you know and human. Now this was a big church with many young people and there were several pretty girls in the congregation. In fact, the pastor's daughter was Miss Tennessee in the Miss America Pageant that year. However, this girl was different. She was more than pretty she was beautiful with a radiance of Madonna. The tailored blue silk pillbox hat was firmly perched on her perfectly groomed coiffeur and face with brown eyes, dimples and perpetual smile. At glances I saw her whisper to her friends with a silent giggle. A restless toddler sitting in front of her turned around and waved to her. She smiled, waved back and patted his hand. I don't recall a word of the sermon or who sat beside me.

As Methodists often do, once the final "A-men" is said they are out of there. I was moved out the back door with the flow as I saw the blue pillbox hat exit out the side door. Kindly greeters shook my hand and invited me to come back. One mentioned I might like to attend the JOY CLASS, a Sunday School Class for Young Adult singles. Ms. Turley was the teacher. I had actually been to the class back when I was a medical student.

Two weeks later I visited the JOY CLASS. I would have been there a week earlier but I had been on duty at the hospital at that time. Sure enough, there she was Jeanette Skinner – this time wearing a large wide-brimmed black hat and looking radiant. She and others greeted me as a visitor without any obvious priority. While I was seemingly just like the others to her she was special to me. I must have blushed like a teenager. I soon learned she treated everyone the same, never pretentious or flirtatious. She was the proverbial Southern Lady – not Southern Belle - but a Southern Lady.

Of course I became a part of the JOY CLASS and attended regularly. These were my kind of people and I went to the extra-church activities where we tended to "hang" (we used this word long before the millennials) and move together. Picnics, concerts, holiday parties, swim parties, etc. were fun things the group experienced while serving the church. Lifetime friendships were made. Jeanette tended to cluster with the girls. They liked her. She was funny and at times created outbursts of female laughter. At times she and I chatted briefly about nonspecific things. I was concerned about a couple of the handsome and charismatic young men who were obviously trying to make advances. Like a poker player she gave them no hint of priority, to my delight. She remained a bright, poised and independent female in complete control at all times.

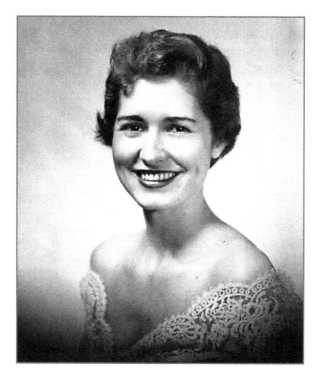

FIG. 9-B: Jeanette when we first met in 1956

After a few weeks of this JOY CLASS togetherness, I began to feel maybe Jeanette was starting to like me a little. I gathered enough courage to ask her for a date.

"Just you and me!" I said.

"I'd love to!" she promptly replied, to my utter delight.

Our first date was on Tuesday, July 31, 1956. We had dinner at the Piccadilly Cafeteria in downtown Memphis on Main St., a place that catered to the moviegoers. Then we went to the beautiful Overton Park in midtown to attend a free concert under the stars at The Overton Park Shell (now called the Levitt Shell). The Memphis Sympathy performed a variety of classical, semi-classical and poplar pieces under the direction of Noel Gilbert. In our scrapbook today I have the program where I had written in bold letters across the top, "I LOVE JEANETTE" **(FIG. 9-C)**. When I passed it to her she looked at it, smiled, put it in her purse and grasped my hand. During dessert after the concert we chatted to get to know each other better. The second date was to a movie and the third was a Jazz concert at the Overton Park Shell on August 21, 1956.

FIG. 9-C: Program of concert we attended on our first date (My handwritten note at top).

Before you ask, we had our first kiss on our third date, saying goodnight at the door of her apartment. Now you want to hear more. Well, you know, I'm a very old person (84 years) and can't remember everything – and besides, you don't need to know anyway. We had a lot of dates **(FIG. 9-D)**.

The next year we were together at every opportunity. Jeanette was sympathetic to my limited financial status and $25 a month salary. She made much more as the Executive Secretary of Slumber Products Co. but never embarrassed me by offering to pay. We both had inexpensive tastes and interests, so money was never an issue with us. We were happy with a lot of free stuff. As a resident at Le Bonheur Children's Hospital I received free meals and a pass for one guest a week in the cafeteria. This was often the site of a date when I was on duty. Jeanette once proudly told her roommate, "We're having dinner at that French restaurant, "Le Bonheur."

We started an event that lasted a lifetime. On Valentine's Day we went together to Walgreen's Greeting Card section, each searched through the cards; I selected one for her and she one for me, handed our selections to each other, read them, thanked each other, placed the cards back on the rack and left hand-in-hand. We considered this event as our protest against the high cost of greeting cards. Once Jeanette said, "You shouldn't have selected such an expensive card."

She loved her family in nearby Brownsville and recalled some of the best times of her life at home with her three sisters and parents and with Sunday dinner at her grandmother's house with a lot of relatives. We found we both liked families, children, movies, gardening, concerts, music, beautiful homes, Methodists and Republicans. She had a passion for dance and dancing and was a superb ballroom dancer. I despised dancing and stumbled on the dance floor. I liked to travel and she found it an inconvenience, preferring to stay home. In Memphis she shared an apartment, and later a house, with three roommates and travelled to work by city bus.

I never on bended knee asked Jeanette to marry me. If I had she probably would have laughed and told me to stop getting my pants dirty. On many occasions I told her I loved her and that I wanted to marry her. She in turn showed her love for me and told me "yes" she wanted to marry me. Our friends and family knew without formal announcement.

A cloud hovered over us. I had been drafted for two years of service in the U. S, Army to begin July 1, 1957. I would spend six weeks of basic training learning to march, salute, shoot guns, etc. at Ft. Sam Houston in San Antonio, TX, and then I would be sent to a permanent post for the remainder of the time. My problem was that most of the inductees were being sent to Korea to phase out the war, and I would be in the high priority group as single and a physician. We decided to await my assignment in mid-August 1957 before deciding on a wedding date.

In San Antonio I was abruptly changed from Dr. Hughes to Captain Hughes, from scrubs to Army green, kaki and dress blue uniforms, from stethoscopes and otoscopes to guns and compasses, from on call every third night to no on call at night, and from a stipend of $25 a month to a salary of $4,800 a year. I was miserable because I missed Jeanette. Texting, cell phones, iPads, email and internet had not been invented. A first class letter took 5 to 7 days to reach Memphis and a phone call cost about three dollars. My thoughts became fixed on mid-August and my permanent assignment. I became more and more convinced I would be sent overseas.

In typical Army style our class graduation was held on the Parade Grounds and we each stepped forward to receive our orders (assignment). I did not open mine until I got back to my room in the BOQ (Bachelor Officers Quarters). When I saw the word MARYLAND I shouted for joy. I wasn't sure where Frederick, Maryland was located and exactly what Ft. Detrick was all about and why I was also assigned to Walter Reed Army Medical Center in Washington, but that didn't matter. I was assigned stateside and I rushed to call Jeanette to tell her so. I then went to a jeweler and bought a solitary diamond ring and sent it to her special delivery. I knew exactly what she liked because we had discussed it earlier. I was ordered to go directly to Ft. Detrick for top-secret clearance and to receive further orders.

I was able to get sufficient leave to be in Memphis a few days before the wedding on November 24, 1957, to help with arrangements and activities for the wedding and to move Jeanette to Maryland. We packed her stuff into a U-Haul rental trailer and hid it for a quick getaway to Maryland after the wedding. Much of the cargo was her favorite plants that she just couldn't leave behind. I had only 3 days left and so we had our honeymoon in route from Memphis to Washington.

The wedding at the First Methodist Church was beautiful and unforgettable. Jeanette as a bride coming down the same isle I had looked across to discover her a year and a half earlier was more beautiful than ever before. **(FIG. 9-E)** When our pastor and friend, Dr. Roy Williams, said, "I now pronounce you man and wife," a new and wonderful life began for me. As ecstatic as I was I had no idea of how wonderful the rest of my life would be.

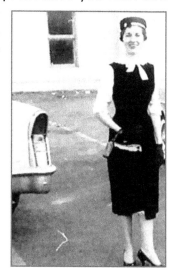

FIG. 9-D: Jeanette on date at church wearing blue silk pillbox hat.

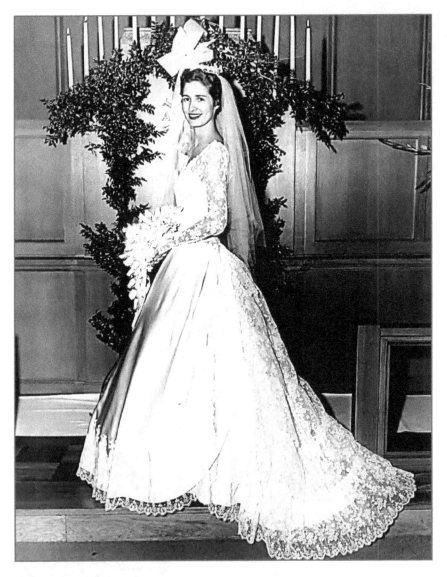

FIG. 9-E: Jeanette the Bride on November 24, 1957, at First Methodist Church, Memphis.

CHAPTER 10
Ft. Detrick and Walter Reed Army Medical Center

My two years at Ft. Detrick in Frederick, Maryland were unique, to say the least. Some background is necessary to fully understand the circumstances.

During World War II the National Academy of Sciences (NAS) reviewed the feasibility of biological ("Germ") warfare and in 1942 recommended that steps be taken to reduce the vulnerability of the United States to biological warfare (BW) attack. Of concern was the potential use by foreign nations of highly infectious organisms and toxic chemicals to attack and kill Americans. In 1943 the **U. S. Army Biological Warfare Laboratories (USBWL)** and pilot plant centers were established at Camp Detrick, in Frederick, MD, nestled in the foothills of the Catoctin Mountains only 60 miles from Washington, DC. The official policy of the United States at that time was to first deter the use of biological warfare against our country and secondarily to retaliate if deterrence failed.

Over the next decade intensive biological warfare research was undertaken using a variety of highly pathogenic bacteria and viruses at Camp Detrick, first overseen by the pharmaceutical executive George W. Merck and by Dr. Ira L. Baldwin, Professor of Bacteriology, at the University of Wisconsin. It was said that from

1945 to 1955 more than 1,600 German and Austrian scientists and engineers were recruited for biological warfare research, including aircraft design and missile technology. In competition for scientists were Great Britain, France and the Soviet Union, also developing BW capability. The BW project was shrouded in secrecy similar to the Manhattan Project in Oak Ridge, Tennessee, and was not made known to the public until four months after VJ (Victory in Japan) Day.

On 20 June 1956, a year before I arrived at Ft. Detrick, a new program named the **United States Army Medical Unit (USAMU)** was established as an additional and separate facility under the jurisdiction of the **Walter Reed Army Medical Center (WRAMC)**. The purpose was to develop defensive measures against biological agents, as opposed to weapons development. The name Camp Detrick was changed to Ft. Detrick. The first **USAMU** commander was **Col. William D. Tigertt,** a Pathologist from the **Walter Reed Army Institute for Research (WRAIR)** in Washington.

Tigertt quickly and effectively established his "Walter Reed Unit" in the midst of Ft. Detrick with the mission to develop defense for Americans against organisms known to be used for biological warfare, in conjunction with the scientists at Ft. Detrick. His command included a headquarters building, a free-standing 15 bed hospital and clinic designated as **Ward 200 of Walter Reed Army Hospital**, and portions of Ft. Detrick research laboratories, including partial use of the now notorious "Building 470". Research projects were targeted and included collaborative efforts with the elaborate basic science disciplines at Ft. Detrick for development of vaccines against *Bacillus anthracis* (the cause of anthrax), *Francisella tularensis* (the cause of tularemia or "rabbit fever") and Venezuela Equine Encephalitis Virus, among other projects. Top-secrete clearance was required for all the staff.

By the time I arrived at Ft. Detrick in August, 1957, a superb core team of senior, nationally- known scientists and clinical investigators in the fields of Infectious Diseases and Microbiology had been amassed under Tigertt's command to undertake the necessary transitional studies in animals and man. All were doctorate level M.D., PhD or both, with ranks of Colonel or equal from career U.S. Army, Navy, National Institutes of Health, U S. Public Health Service ranks; or, under contract from academic institutions in nearby Baltimore (Johns Hopkins U., U. Maryland) and Washington (Georgetown U, George Washington U.) and elsewhere (Ohio State U. College of Medicine). **(FIG. 10-A)**

I, and three similar novices, all physicians drafted at the completion of residency training, arrived within a month of each other and held the rank of Captain. Over ensuing months an additional four Captains joined the group. We functioned very much like Fellows in Infectious Diseases in traditional academic programs working in both research labs as well translational clinical research projects. We were also assigned to limited clinical service at Ward 200 for the care of Ft. Detrick employees.

Although my involvement with the WRAMC group at Ft. Detrick occurred more than 50 years ago a few notes are jotted down below about those with whom I worked most closely.

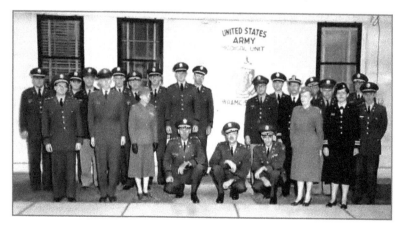

FIG. 10-A: Walter Reed Army Medical Unit, Ft. Detrick, MD – 1957
Col. Edwin Overholt, Col. Alice Clark, Col. Collin Vorde Brugge, Col. William Tigertt, Dr. Martha Ward, Col. William S. Gochenaur, Col. Robert G. Yaeger, Capt. Richard Hornick, Capt. Kenneth Vosti, Capt. William Burmeister, Capt. Walter Hughes, Capt. Aaron Meislin, Capt. Ted Salzman.

Some memory notes:

Col. William D. Tigertt: MD, Baylor U. College of Medicine (Internal Medicine and Pathology).

- My Commanding Officer.

- Tall, slender with mustache. Intensive worker, scholar, administrator, researcher; independent and impersonal; fair; expected perfection.

- Wife Helen took liking to my bride Jeanette and held luncheon at the Commanding Officer's home in her honor and to introduce her to officers' wives.

- Later: promoted to General; retired to become Professor of Medicine and Professor of Pathology and Associate Chairman, Dept. Pathology, University of Maryland Medical School.

Col. Colin F. Vorder Brugge: MD University of Tennessee College of Medicine (Pathology).

- Second in Command to Tigertt; also prominent role in Office of Surgeon General in Washington; charismatic, interactive, leader, research-oriented.

- From a prominent Memphis military-medicine family. Befriended Jeanette and me due in part to Memphis ties.

- One afternoon soon after I arrived he called and said his young daughter (6-7 yr.) might be getting measles. (I was the only Pediatrician on post at the time). She had just developed fever and rash and some other children on post had measles. Did I have any suggestions? I told him I would stop by his house and see her on my way home. She had high fever and rash, but no coryza, cough and conjunctivitis (almost always present with measles). With the red maculopapular measles-like rash were a few petechiae and her neck was difficult to flex. Despite the strong exposure to measles the diagnosis of meningococcal meningitis, a rapid-ly fatal infection was possible. I felt like a Tennessee country boy with mud on his shoes when I told the Colonel I thought a diagnostic spinal tap was indicated, but if he wanted an-other opinion I would contact a Pediatrician at WRAH in Washington. He and his wife asked me to proceed with the spinal tap. They realized the importance of timing.

In a treatment room on Ward 200, with the aid of a nurse (Col. Alice Clark, RN, the highest ranking women in the U.S. Army at the time) I performed a spinal tap that re-vealed 15 white blood cells, slightly low glucose level and negative Gram stain of the spinal fluid. These results were borderline, not diagnostic but did not exclude the diagnosis. I admitted her to an isolation room on Ward 200 and started intravenous antibiotics empirically for meningitis.

By morning when I came to the ward and office I felt all eyes were on stupid me for doing a spinal tap on a child with measles. In late afternoon I received a call from Dr. Martha Ward, a senior researcher, who had personally supervised the culture of the spinal fluid, saying the culture was grow-ing *Neisseria meningitidis*, the bacterium that causes men-ingitis. Within a week the child was well at home.

This was another time when I thought the good Lord was looking out for me.

- Later: Vorder Brugge was promoted to Major <u>General</u> and Commander of Research and Development in the Office of the Surgeon General.

Col. Edwin L. Overholt: MD University of Iowa Medical Center and Fitzsimmons Hospital

- Superb internist dedicated to work, very likeable, interac-tive, teacher, Korean War hero (Silver Star for Gallantry in action; Legion of Merit); VIP Ward Consultant at WRAH for President Eisenhower, Vice President Nixon, General Douglas MacArthur and others.

- My immediate supervisor. The other Captains and I were under his direction.
- Main research at Ft. Detrick was tularemia project and vaccine trials.
- Later: up for promotion to General but left Army to become Director of Education at Gundersen Medical Center, Clinical Professor of Medicine at U. of Wisconsin, Madison and Clinical Professor of Medicine U. Iowa, Iowa City. Died 2006.

Dr. Martha K. Ward: PhD, U.S. Public Health Service, CDC, Georgetown U., George Washington U.

- Internationally renowned Microbiologist/ Bacteriologist/ Immunologist.
- Research lab at Ft. Detrick and consultant in operation of clinical microbiology laboratories.
- Prolific publications
- Later: Died 1994.

Col. William S. Gochenaur: DVM. Dept. Veterinary Bacteriology and Special Operations Branch, Walter Reed Army Institute of Research

- Expert Leptospirosis

Col. Robert Yeager, PhD:

- Later: Professor Dept. Tropical Medicine, School of Public Health, and Professor of Medicine, Dept. Medicine, Tulane University School of Medicine, New Orleans, LA.

Col. Alice Clark: RN; Director of Nurses at WRAMU, Ward 200.

- Excellent nurse, Korean War hero, dedicated to service, co-operative with all.
- Highest ranking nurse, and woman, in the U. S. Army at this time.

THE CAPTAINS: Two-year Service Inductees: from residency to Ft. Detrick:

Capt. Richard B. Hornick: MD (Internal Medicine – Johns Hopkins University School of Medicine)

- We shared office.
- Wife Adele was a friend of Jeanette's.
- Later: became Professor and Chairman, Dept. Medicine University of Rochester School of Medicine. Elected to Institute of Medicine, more than 300 publications. Died in 2011 of cancer.

Capt. Kenneth Vosti: MD (Internal Medicine – Stanford University College of Medicine)

- We shared office
- Met his wife Anne in Frederick where she was a student at Hood College. Married soon after Jeanette and I married.
- Later: Professor of Medicine, Stanford University College of Medicine; Emeritus Faculty, Academic Council, meritorious career at Stanford U. where he and Anne still live.

Capt. R. William Burmeister: MD (Internal Medicine – St. Louis University School of Medicine)

- Later: Infectious Diseases Practice, St. Louis

Capt. Walter T. Hughes: MD (Pediatrics – University of Tennessee College of Medicine)

- See **APPENDIX II** *Curriculum vitae.*

Capt. Aaron G. Meislin: MD *(Pediatrics – New York University School of Medicine; Bellevue* Hospital.)

- Wife Monica, friend of Jeanette.

- Later: Pediatrics, New York City; staff Bellevue Hospital and NYU Hospital; Board of Directors NY County Medical Society; died 2013.

Capt. Theodore Salzman: MD

Note of interest: Another Ft. Detrick Captain who arrived after my group had left was **Ralph D. Feigin, M.D.,** who became an icon in the field of Pediatric Infectious Diseases, and eventually President, Baylor College of Medicine, Houston.

My work at Ft. Detrick was primarily associated with the evaluation of a vaccine against *Francisella tularensis,* an extremely virulent bacterium that causes the potentially fatal disease Tularemia in animals and man. It was well known among nations as a more ideal biological warfare agent that could be dispersed in air, water and food and would be highly infective. Because we were in the era of the Cold War with Russia, and the U.S. War Department had learned that the Russians were immunizing thousands of their population against tularemia, some priority was focused on tularemia vaccine at Ft, Detrick. Ampules of the Russian vaccine were obtained "indirectly" and brought to Ft. Detrick for analysis (Heinz Eiglesbach; Paul Kadull) and evaluation.

The initial studies were done in the laboratory utilizing animal experiments with Rhesus monkeys carried out in state-of-the-art animal facilities developed for use of highly infectious agents and with limited access. Now declassified and published descriptions of Building 470 serve as an example of Ft. Detrick facilities. Vividness in my memory causes me to comment further. Building 470, also known as "The Tower", "Anthrax Tower" and "Pilot Plant' has been the topic of many Ft. Detrick stories, some true and some fiction. The seven-story structure was the tallest on post and its size and shape was determined by the fact that it housed two 2,500-gallon fermenters, three-stories high, extending on top of the first two floors. The entire building was hermetically sealed under negative pressure. The top floor was occupied by powerful air-handling systems to maintain the integrity of infection control. The fermentation tanks were used for the production of *Bacillus anthracis, Franciscella tularensis and Brucella suis.* Unrelated to any function, the outside of the structure was designed to include false windows and windowsills for disguise or camophlage as an office building or barracks. The bottom two floors were designed with facilities for scientists to shower and change clothes to germ-protective garbs.

In 1958, while I (and Jeanette) lived on post, a large spill occurred in Building 470 when a technician trying to pry open a valve on one of the fermenter tanks accidently released 2,000 gallons of liquid *Bacillus anthracis* (anthrax) culture. The design of the building and safety system contained the spill to one room and no contamination of Ft. Detrick occurred. The technician and other exposed employees were managed at Ward 200 and none became ill.

The tularemia vaccine animal studies were done in great part by the Captains, including Dick Hornick, Ken Vosti, Bill Burmeister and myself. With all due modesty, I was essential to the experiments. Blood samples for testing were required daily or more often. These Rhesus monkeys brought from the wild to Ft. Detrick were easily capable of biting off a finger, so gaining access to vein was very difficult. As a Pediatrician I had become skilled at drawing blood from the femoral vein near the groin in tiny babies and was able to do so in the monkeys restrained by two animal technicians on a board device. Sampling from other venous sites was almost impossible. At times while drawing blood in the wee hours of the morning, I wondered if Tigertt with his meticulous planning ahead might not have brought a Pediatrician into the group just to draw blood samples.

My indelible memory of the laboratory is entry and exit during the snowy winters in Maryland. In some experiments I would need to do a procedure as often as every 8 hours around the clock. From my office or home I would walk to a building fenced and guarded, enter a locker room, remove **all** clothes, watch, ring, etc., don a protective garment, often of cold impervious paper, gloves, mask and cap, and move through a transitional pressure room to the lab maintained at continuous negative pressure. To exit the entire garb was removed and left discarded in the lab, leaving me stark naked in front of caged monkeys and coworkers. I then went through a barrier into the shower room for total soapy shower hair to toes, through an air dryer, processed items taken out through ultraviolet light cabinets (x 10 min); then I went through the transitional pressure barrier to locker room, to re-dress and exit. Still damp from shower and hitting the freezing night on the walk home was memorable. Going through this ritual every 8 hours for several days or so left one very clean with red chapped skin. To think of myself as a soldier serving my country brought little solace, but a Purple Heart seemed reasonable.

The monkey experiments showed the tularemia vaccine to be effective and safe, even when immunized animals were challenged with *Francisella tularensis* by the respiratory route. After thorough review of research protocols by The Armed Forces Epidemiological Board, several governmental committees, and academic Consultants, clinical trials of the vaccine in humans were undertaken.

The clinical trials under Col. Tigertt's command from Ft. Detrick with Col. Overholt and his Captains (Vosti, Hornick, Burmeister and Hughes) were started at the Ohio State Penitentiary in Columbus, OH. A contract with Dr. Samuel Saslaw, Professor of Medicine, at Ohio State University School of Medicine provided local collaboration.

Up to a point the tularemia project at Ohio State Petitionary was classified as top-secret and I was required to remove all identification related to Ft. Detrick and the Army, to rent an automobile and drive from Frederick to Columbus, rent an apartment near the college campus, and report for duty at a specific entrance of the prison at a designated hour. Because the assignment was expected to last several weeks or months, we Captains were allowed to bring our wives with us if we wished. Jeanette and I had been married only a few months and of course I very much wished her to be with me. The day after my arrival the project was announced in prison and local newspapers. I must note here that during my off-duty time Jeanette and I had many enjoyable times together in Columbus, a city much like Memphis.

After full disclosure prisoners were allowed to volunteer for the project to receive the vaccine and later be challenged by *F.*

tularensis by the respiratory route. The number of qualified volunteers far exceeded the number needed for the study. The men in groups of six were admitted to a ward in the prison hospital where I and the other Captains rotated in teams of two living in continuously, 24/7, with the men. As we moved from phase to phase of the clinical trials, a few other Captains came from Ft. Detrick.

From group to group the volunteers were remarkably similar: all had committed felonies including murder, robbery, embezzlement, etc.; were between 21 and 35 years old, had volunteered in order to escape prison boredom or to pay retribution for their crimes, or both. Their only benefit from participation was to stay on the hospital ward and watch television. They sat and watched the small, black and white TV from the first flicker in the morning until the snowy end at midnight. Their favorite program was "Queen for a Day", bringing some to tears. Male nurses from the prison hospital served our patients and aided us as needed. Our meals were served along with the volunteers and we came to know our patients very well with no fear from their presence. One of the hospital inmate trustees, a "nurse-anesthesiologist," was the infamous Dr. Sam Shepherd, an osteopathic physician from Cleveland, OH convicted of killing his wife. He was into bodybuilding and was well liked by other inmates in some circles but not in others. Our study progressed well and none of the subjects suffered any significant adverse effects, a point about we were most concerned. Eventually, the results were reported in medical journals by Saslow, Overholt, *et al.*

Returning to Frederick I had no idea of the truly remarkable event yet to be experienced. Within a year I had married my precious Jeanette, left for the first time my native Tennessee, been made a part of icons of my profession, located in a most exciting area (Washington) of the world and had leisure time to continually increase my love and devotion to Jeanette. Our lives expanded from the southeast to the northeast, with weekend explorations of all the sights of Washington, DC, Baltimore, Annapolis, Ocean City, New York City, Gettysburg and Philadelphia. I had even come to own an adult toy from boyhood dreams – a 1954 MG Roadster sports car with headlights on fenders and cloth top, purchased on a Baltimore used car for $500. In addition to the exciting surrounding attractions, Jeanette also loved the quiet weekends in Frederick.

Much can be said about Frederick — a paradox to Ft. Detrick. From Jeanette's view Frederick was a tranquil, old, beautiful small town, where people came to know each other and live together as a small town. Of Frederick **John Greenleaf Whittier** once wrote:

"Up from the meadows rich with corn,
   Clear in the cool September morn,
The clustered spires of Frederick stand,
   Green-walled by the hills of Maryland."

We often visited the calm beautiful Culler Lake in midtown where families of ducks flocked to visitors. The only restaurant for a special time out was at the local hotel. Alternatives were the Officers' Clubs at Ft. Detrick, Walter Reed Medical Center and Bethesda Naval Center — all within an hour's drive. Jeanette liked them all. An advantage to Bethesda was that when I called for reservations for Captain and Mrs. Hughes we were placed a notch higher, because the rank of Captain in the Navy was equal to Colonel in the Army.

A special occasion occurred in the summer of 1958 when Jeanette with beaming smiles announced she was with child. I was overjoyed. We both wanted children in our lives. This was the highlight of our year. When asked, we both replied that we had no preference as to boy or girl. However, I felt Jeanette would really like to have a little girl.

The excellent Obstetricians at WRAH provided state of the art prenatal care. An Army car and driver took her from home to clinic and she never missed a visit, took every vitamin tablet and bought Dr. Spock's book (hard cover version) on childcare.

One weekend in mid-March, 1959 Jeanette and I took a long ride in my MG sports car, with convertible top down, across the beautiful Maryland springtime countryside, driving over hills and vales in a vehicle with the comfort of an Army tank. Later in the day some fleeting abdominal pains were noticed and we were near the time for delivery. I took her to the OB Clinic at WRAH. The Obstetrician said she was not yet in labor but he would her admit her for the night and examine her in the morning. He said regulations would not allow me to stay with her and that I should go back home and he would call me if needed. So, I drove back to Frederick arriving in our on-post apartment after 11:00 PM.

Sometime after midnight on March 19, 1959 I was awakened by a phone call from Jeanette. She said in a somewhat groggy voice,

"We have a little girl."

"Are you all right?" I asked.

"I'm OK."

"Is the baby OK?"

"Yes, she's beautiful!"

"How much did she weigh?"

"Thirteen pounds and seven ounces!" she answered.

My heart sank. I knew that 90% infants weighing more than 13 pounds at birth are Diabetic.

"I'm on my way".

Some background information is in order.

In 1959 throughout the United States outbreaks of infection caused by *Staphylococcus aureus* penicillin-resistant, were occurring in hospitals and causing fatalities in newborn nurseries.

The nursery at Walter Reed Army Hospital, as in other leading medical centers established strict guidelines to prevent infection in infants. Entry to the nursery was limited so that fathers and other relatives were not allowed to have contact with their infants until several days after birth.

A local policy at Walter Reed was that the mother, not the doctor, would be the first to tell the father of the birth. Essentially, by bedside-side phone when awake after delivery, the mother would tell the father by phone about the birth. It was here that Jeanette, still groggy, had reversed the figures from the real values of Carla's birth measurements of 7 pounds, 13 ounces and 22 inches in length. **(FIG. 10-B)**

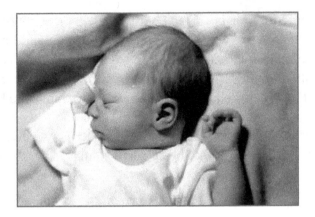

FIG. 10-B: Carla, soon after birth.

WALTER REED ARMY HOSPITAL
WALTER REED ARMY MEDICAL CENTER
WASHINGTON, D.C.

HOSPITAL BIRTH CERTIFICATE

This Certifies that   CARLA LYNNE HUGHES

was born in WALTER REED ARMY HOSPITAL, WASHINGTON, D.C.

on the   NINETEENTH   day of   MARCH   A. D. 19 59

The official registration of this birth has been made with the Health Department of the

District of Columbia.

HOSPITAL REGISTER No. 5192 007

For The Commander

FIG. 10-C: Carla Lynne Hughes, born on 19 Mar 1959, Walter Reed Army Hospital, Washington, DC.

It was some three days before I could actually hold our little baby while Jeanette had contact immediately after birth. The importance of <u>immediate</u> "bonding" by parent and child is somewhat dispelled by Carla, because some 50 years later I cannot imagine a closer and more lovable lifetime relationship with my daughter.

We brought our baby and exuberant mother back to our new quarters at Ft. Detrick. Both grandmothers were blessed. Carla was born on my mother's birthday and Jeanette's mother came to Fredrick to help us during this important time.

It was some three months after Carla's birth that we ended our stay in Maryland and returned to Tennessee.

NOTE: **"A Ft. Detrick Serendipity Ditty:"**

More than 30 years after we left Ft. Detrick Jeanette and I were having dinner at a local restaurant where seating was not ideal and the odor of tobacco smoke drifted to our no- smoking section. Jeanette detested tobacco smoke and among other comments said, "If I could I would destroy all the tobacco in the world. It kills people, it is good for nothing and besides it's nasty." I began to think about what she said and recalled a large research program in Plant Pathology at Ft. Detrick during my tour there. The intent was to destroy crops as a part of biological warfare. I was in no position to become involved in research to destroy tobacco, but the idea of genetic engineering to develop bacteria that could destroy tobacco plants was intriguing. So, I wrote a novel called **The Last Leaf,** published in 2003 (Writer's Club Press, New York) in which seven Ft. Detrick scientists secretly used hidden labs to create, develop and disperse an anthrax-like organism that accomplished the destruction of every vestige of tobacco in the world. The subsequent events made an interesting science fiction story.

FIG. 10-D: Walter and Jeanette 33 years after leaving Ft. Detrick.

CHAPTER 11

Back Home to Cleveland

On 8 Aug 1959 I received an Honorable Discharge from the Army of the United States after two years of service to our country. It was now time for me to enter another major change in my life, but this time unlike heretofore I was not alone. I had my dear Jeanette, precious Carla, two used cars, about $4,000 in the bank and no debts.

At age 29 years I would return to my hometown of Cleveland, TN to enter private practice of Pediatrics. My mother and sister Katherine still lived there. This move was not from a recent decision but rather from a commitment I had made more than two years earlier as a Resident in Pediatrics in Memphis. In fact its origin may go back even further. Prior to the time when Dr. Ettledorf said "Hughes, you should write up this case for the medical journal," I had thought of myself as one going into private practice in Cleveland, where the services of a Pediatrician had been sought for years earlier.

In Memphis I came to know and like Dr. Hayes Mitchell, a fellow resident during the second year of residency. Hayes was married. He and his wife Geneva had me to their apartment for dinner. Hayes had served his time in the military and was looking for a place to set up practice when he finished his training. One of my concerns about Cleveland was my survival as a solo practice because of the large population to be served. I suggested he and Geneva consider going to Cleveland while I was in the Army and that I would return and join him two years later. They visited Cleveland, liked it and the plan was set. As expected, from the first day on Hayes saw patients from dawn to dusk and even later.

By the time I returned to Cleveland Hayes was exhausted. Because our new office space was not finished, he left at my suggestion on a two-week vacation soon after I arrived and I used his office to cover the practice. On my first day I saw more than 20 patients and the number increased thereafter.

During the second week, with waiting room packed I had an emergency call from the hospital to see an infant with jaundice due to Rh incompatibility. An exchange blood transfusion was needed immediately if the life could be saved. This procedure to exchange the baby's blood with that of a donor had never been done in Cleveland, although it was well established as the treatment that should be done for this condition. So, I had to put together trays of tubing, syringes, pumps and connectors to start the procedure, which I had done frequently at Le Bonheur.

I finished the procedure at about 7:00 pm and decided to go back to the office and close up. Surprisingly, four patients with weary parents were still in our waiting room. I got home at about 10:00 pm. Subsequently, I was faced with wall-to-wall patients every day. Lest you be misled to thinking of a superdoc Pediatrician, I must tell you that was clearly not the case. The vast majority of patients regularly seen had only minor illnesses or none at all. Giving immunization shots, treating colds and diarrhea, dealing with feeding problems for children not eating well or those eating too much; physical exams for school, evaluating behavior problems and parents' concerns about over active, under active, overweight, underweight, over achiever, under achiever, and grade-failing children filled my days.

Jeanette and I were able to rent a two-bedroom house from one of the local General Practitioners, Dr. Claude Taylor, my mother's doctor and a member of our church. It was located two blocks from my mother and sister and about a 5- minutes' drive from our office. Despite many offers for start-up loans I did not commit to the purchase of a house or office. My expected income from practice was about $15,000 for the first year with full partnership to follow. I had already failed Millie's rule to "wait until you can pay before you buy," in the purchase of our yellow and white Buick. However, the $500 for the 1954 MG roadster was paid in cash. Incidentally, the vintage cloth top sports car with "up North" license plate did not go unnoticed in the hospital parking lot.

It didn't take long for us to settle in because I was still remembered by many people in town. We joined the First Methodist Church where our baby Carla was christened. Jeanette and I had dinner at the homes of my old friends. Our little 2,000 sq. ft. house limited any big social functions. We really preferred to be alone when I had any time away from work. Our favorite "date" was to drive 30 miles to Brainerd, a suburb of Chattanooga, have dinner at a small restaurant there and go to a movie, with popcorn.

Life in Cleveland was of course quite different from life in Maryland and Washington, but Jeanette and I loved both. She was totally devoted to doting over her baby Carla, sharing her with my mother and making a home for us. Emerging early on here was a single fetish of Jeanette that persisted for more than half a century, and I can think of no others. She was of the obsession that her husband and children should be home at a specified time for dinner. She always prepared a delicious hot meal for us all to sit and enjoy. Explanations that I had to see a sick child in the Emergency Room, or that I still had patients to be seen in the office, were reluctantly acceptable (if I called earlier to inform her). I soon came to appreciate her feelings by realizing she had never been associated with doctors, nurses and the medical field. However, as time went on she became oriented to the problems of practice and I to those of a dedicated wife.

You must realize my time in private practice in 1960 was different from that of today. There were no cell phones, texting, email, computers or internet. I had to stay near a line-connected phone at all times I was on call (every day and every other night). Patients were accustomed to calling their doctors at home as well as the office. Jeanette soon heard my routine answers to many questions such as what to do for earache, diarrhea, fever, vomiting, etc. So, when she answered the phone and I was not available, she would often give advice saying, "This is what he usually does ..." As a concerned mother she may have been more convincing than I, because I later received good comments from patients about her helpfulness. Practice in the office was somewhat different from today. There were no Nurse Practitioners, Nurse Physician Assistants, and the office RN was much more limited in what she could do.

We had no business office. One woman served as the receptionist, secretary and billing agent. Most people paid at the time of the visit and insurance was a rare item. I cannot recall any patient who did not received the treatment needed, regardless of ability to pay. The well-stocked cabinet of drug samples from drug companies would be dubbed today as "promotional" and discouraged, and the pharmaceutical Rep a lobbyist. I can testify that these resources were at times life saving and were immediately available, in contrast to present-day government bureaucracy.

Soon after I arrived in Cleveland Hayes and I moved into a new Clinic building at 3315 Broad St. (changed to 90 Broad St.) where we leased office space. The Clinic included the offices of two Obstetricians, a Dentist and a free-standing Pharmacy. Serendipitous details are footnoted at the end of this chapter.

Great news came in the spring of 1960 when Jeanette announced we were going to have another baby. This brought joy to my heart. We had often mentioned to each other that a family of three children would be ideal. When we were asked what gender we were hoping for we both responded that either would fine and that we had no preferences. However, deep down I really favored a boy. I really wanted to have a son, if not now we would try again later.

On the evening of October 25 Jeanette and I attended a formal social event at the Cleveland Country Club. It was a dinner and dance and Jeanette was within a few days of the expected time for delivery. We were seated with Dr. and Mrs. Gilbert Varnell along with some other friends. Gilbert was Jeanette's Obstetrician and shared clinic office space with Hayes and myself. Gilbert had the last dance of the evening with Jeanette. After we arrived at home Jeanette began with early labor pains. I called Gilbert and his answering service informed me his partner, Dr. John Rogness, who had also seen Jeanette, was now on call for the night. John met us in the ER at Bradley County Hospital and admitted her to the delivery suite. Here, in contrast to Walter Reed Hospital, I was able to stay with her until she went into the delivery room. Thereafter, I waited in the nearby Doctor's Lounge until John came in and told me in the traditional fashion that I was the father of a healthy baby boy. When I reached Jeanette's room she was sound asleep and did not awaken for a couple of hours. When she awoke I was able to tell her what she had told me when Carla was born, "We have a baby—".

"I don't remember, I've been asleep," she said while half awake.

"It's a boy! We have our Greg."

"I want to hold him!" was her immediate plea. "He's beautiful! I can't believe we have a little boy.

She was from a family of four girls and no boys.

The next day I brought Carla to the room to see her little brother. She wanted to touch him and pat his hand - a spitin' image of her mother, I thought. From that time on little Greg had two females mothering his every need. I got my chance too.

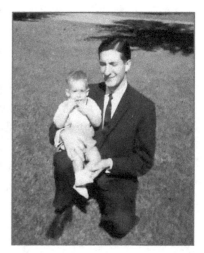

FIG. 11-A:
Greg and Walter in Cleveland.

Despite a thriving practice, a supportive partner and friend in Hayes Mitchell, a modern-state-of-the-art Clinic, a beautiful town and community in which to live with heritage back to Wales, a perfect wife and children, good health, being close to my mother and sister, secure if not lucrative financial future likely, and lifelong friends as neighbors, as well as other blessings, I began to feel something was missing in my life. Unlike any other times in my life, when I thought of future goals to seek, none was there. Accumulation of wealth and property was never a stimulus for Jeanette or me. I was never a depressed person but I just felt a need to accomplish more than I was doing at that time.

After more than a year in Cleveland Jeanette and I were having a weekend "date" at our favorite restaurant in Chattanooga. While I was never a big talker, I must have been less so than usual tonight. Jeanette sensed a problem and as usual came directly to the point.

"You seem sad tonight, Sweetie. Is something troubling you?"

"Well, I have no reason to be sad. In fact I should be happy. Somehow lately I seem to feel I'm just not doing the most of what I could be doing. I work day and night seeing patients knowing that I relieve the suffering of some and help anxious mothers, but I am having no impact on the real problems of medicine. I'm just not very happy with what I do."

"What do you want to do? "

"I think I would like to get into academic medicine to do research and teaching, but that would be totally out of the question here in Cleveland.

"I've thought for some time you have not been all that happy here, so what can we do about it?

You know I'll go wherever you want to go."

For the first time in months I felt a surge of excitement and we talked 'till midnight, forgetting the movie we had planned to attend. At Ft. Detrick I had received some offers to be considered for junior positions in academic institutions. Hornick had gone directly to a fellowship at the University of Maryland and Vosti had returned to Stanford University School of Medicine. Dr. Ettledorf had invited me back to the University of Tennessee College of Medicine for a Fellowship for which he had funding. A change would mean much lower income for years to come, move to a larger city and taking a chance on success.

"I think we should go for it!" was Jeanette's conclusion. And we did.

After some searching I gave up the idea of a fellowship because the Ft. Detrick experience exceeded by far what available fellowships offered. I interviewed for a postdoc position in the Department of Microbiology at Duke University and declined because I would spend a couple of years studying viruses by electron microscopy, less exciting than treating ear infections.

Somehow, I don't recall exactly why, Dr. Alex Steigman, Chairman of the Department of Pediatrics at the University of Louisville School of Medicine invited me to interview for a position of Instructor in Pediatrics, an entry level faculty position, in his department. He was nationally known as a specialist in infectious diseases and was editor and chairman of the American Academy of Pediatrics "Redbook" Committee that established the guidelines for management of infections in children. He seemed to appreciate my Ft. Detrick experience. A job offer with a salary of $14,000 was forthcoming, much more than I had expected for my venture into academic medicine at the time. Moreover, when Jeanette visited Louisville we fell in love the old city on the Ohio River, with beautiful homes and parks, Churchill Downs and horse country, good schools, theater and symphony, and friendly down-to-earth people.

I was tremendously excited about going to Louisville, as was Jeanette, although much of the excitement was probably because of my own. An added bonus was the agreement of my mother and sister to also move to Louisville.

We moved to Louisville in 1961 and I began my new job as Instructor in Pediatrics, absolutely the lowest rung of the faculty ladder, at the University of Louisville School of Medicine.

94

SERENDIPITY DITY FROM CLEVELAND:

FIGURE 11-B below is a Google Earth, present-day rendition, of the site of my childhood in Cleveland, TN described in chapter 6 and shown in **(FIGS. 6A-6C)**. The areas of Johnston Park, the First Methodist Church, The Princess Theater and the Cherokee Hotel are essentially unchanged, except for renovations. I draw your attention to the area of the empty parking lot the site of **3315 (later 90) Broad Street.** The sequence of events at this site is:

1936: residence and the office and showroom of the **HUGHES FUNERAL HOME.**
1939: Walter Sr. dies leaving property to Millie and children.
195?: Millie sells property to Gilbert Varnell.
1958: Building demolished.
1960: New Cleveland Clinic Building opens with offices for:

> Gilbert Varnell, M.D. Obstetrics
> John Rogness, M.D. Obstetrics
> Hayes Mitchell, M.D. Pediatrics
> Walter Hughes, M.D., Pediatrics*
> Vernon (Pete) Bryant, DDS, Dentist
> Pharmacy

2010: Hays Mitchell, M.D. dies.
200?: Cleveland Clinic Building Demolished.

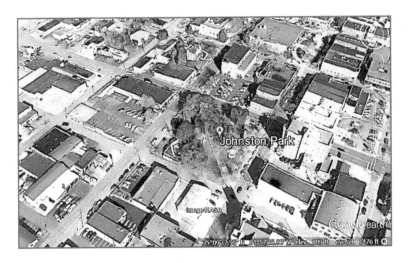

FIG. 11-B: AREA OF JOHNSTON PARK, CLEVELAND TN TODAY (2014, FROM Google Earth) (original address 3315 Broad St. later changed to 90) (Parking lot, upper left); First Methodist Church (lower right); Princess Theater (Middle right, white building); Cherokee Hotel (upper right, brick building).

CHAPTER 12

Louisville

Louisville is an old city, founded in 1778 by George Rogers Clark who named it after King Louis XII of France, making it one of the oldest cities west of the Appalachian Mountains. Some have referred to it as the most northern of southern cities, and others have referred to it as the most southern of northern cities. Located about 100 miles from Cincinnati, Ohio, on the border of Indiana and Kentucky, the area is known as Kentuckiana and is situated at the Falls of the Ohio River. The population of the metropolitan area is about one million people.

At the time of our move in 1961, Louisville was best known for the Kentucky Derby at Churchill Downs, Bluegrass countryside with beautiful horse farms, whiskey distilleries (one-third of all Bourbon produced came from Louisville), tobacco industry (Brown and Williamson; R. J. Reynolds Companies), Louisville Slugger bats and the University of Louisville Cardinals (and Medical School).

Finding a place to live was easy because there were many ideal residential neighborhoods throughout the city and beyond. Purchasing a place to live was a different matter. Despite our financial limitations we found our almost "dream home" on Chadwick Rd., in the suburban Moorgate subdivision. The problem was that we were not able to make the 10% down payment on the enormous purchase of price of $26,000. Coming to our rescue was my little brother Joe, now an unmarried Orthopedic Surgeon in Atlanta, who gave us a second loan of $1,000 for one year.

This was our first home to own (with mortgage) and our lives in Louisville were very happy. Jeanette's creative talent for interior design and decoration kept her focused on transforming our drab Georgian house to a showplace. See chapter 16. Next-door neighbors, the Parnells, were friends for Carla, Jeanette and myself. Little Greg chose to play alone with Matchbox cars rather than play dolls with the Parnell girls and Carla. Several months later my mother and sister moved to Louisville into their own house about five miles from Moorgate, offering Greg and Carla a new playground.

I believe living in Louisville and working at the University of Louisville were more gratifying and enjoyable than almost any part of my professional career. Jeanette, Carla, Greg and I found many things to do- picnics in Cherokee Park, cookouts with friends, Cardinals Basketball, good restaurants, watching Kentucky Derby, visiting beautiful horse farms, time with my mother and sister, a vibrant church family at St. Paul Methodist Church, events on the Ohio River, movies, theater and musicals. My colleagues at work were both respected academic professionals and good friends.

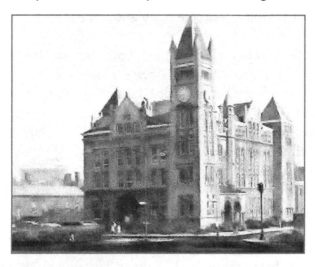

FIG.12-A: Historic Administration Building, School of Medicine, University of Louisville.

Like Louisville, the University of Louisville was also old – founded in 1798. The Louisville Medical Institute was chartered in 1833 and opened in 1837. As with some ten other "medical colleges " in Louisville, the faculty was derived from local practicing physicians, lacked scientific base, attracted large enrollments, prospered financially, and remained separate from the university. I mention this in order to tell you about one of the greatest contributions in the history of American medicine that came solely from a young, meek Louisville school teacher. In a sense he was the founder of the "Academic Medicine" career to which I aspired.

Abraham Flexner was born in 1866 in Louisville, graduated with a Bachelor of Arts degree from Johns Hopkins University at age 19 years and then became an innovative private school teacher in Louisville. Although he had never been inside a medical school, he was selected by the American Medical Association to undertake a study of medical education in the United States. Over a period of two years he personally visited 155 medical schools in the U.S. and Canada, doing his own assessment and often going back later secretly to verify what he been told and shown. The meticulous factual detail was the strength of the famous **Flexner Report** published in 1910 under the aegis of the **Carnegie Foundation**.

In summary, the **Flexner Report** recommended: the <u>closure</u> of 124 of the 155 medical schools (including the Louisville Medical Institute); the training of physicians based on science and factual information; that clinical professors should be full-time positions devoted to teaching and research and barred from all but charity practice; the medical school be a part of a university; and emphasis be placed on small classes, personal attention and hands-on teaching. His report was followed by a wave of reformation in medical education in the United States and Flexner was later called to Europe for further studies on medical education there.

Over the first half of the 20th century, boosted by the **Flexner Report**, the University of Louisville School of Medicine became a progressive and vibrant institution for the training of physicians in compliance with Flexner's recommendations.

At the time of my arrival in 1961 the Department of Pediatrics had a full-time faculty located at the **Louisville General Hospital** (LGH, the city-county 'charity' teaching hospital) with a Newborn Nursery, 30-bed Pediatric ward and outpatient clinics; a **Children's' Hospital** (a privately owned facility staffed by the University of Louisville as a teaching institution), a **Child Evaluation Center** (Falkner, an N.I.H. sponsored research unit) housed next door to LGH and research laboratories in the **Medical Dental Research Facility** in Virology (Steigman) and Biophysical Chemistry (Brodsky). In addition, selected competent Pediatricians in private practice came to the teaching hospitals to volunteer sharing their hands-on experience with students and residents, a decidedly positive effect on training of medical practitioners.

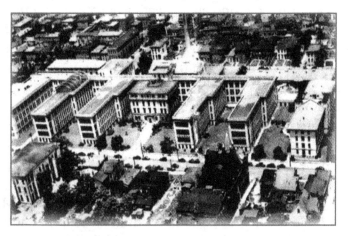

FIG. 12-B: Louisville General Hospital, 500 beds.

My 6 ft. x 9 ft. office at LGH was located adjacent to that of the Chairman, Dr. Alex Steigman, not for any priority because I was the lowest and newest one in the department. Rather, Steigman had contributed his storage closet for my space. My assignments were to attend the outpatient clinics daily to supervise and checkout the students and their patients; manage the weekly Chest Clinic for children with tuberculosis; rotate in the inpatient attending ward rounds with residents and students and give the student lectures on Infant Feeding.

I sensed that my lectures to young unmarried men about infant feeding were failing to create interest. At this time the America Academy of Pediatrics was strongly promoting breast-feeding as preferred over formula feeding for little babies. When I added the concept of "disuse atrophy" to my lectures, ears perked up. I reasoned to the students that in the evolutionary process of nature when organs and tissues are not used they become atrophic, shrink and may fade from the species. Thus, if formula in a bottle replaces the practice of breast-feeding of little babies one might someday expect a world of breast-less women. Subsequently, I noticed in the clinic students had a renewed interest in counseling their parents on breast-feeding. The point to be made here is that I learned early on that humor could be an important component of a lecture.

One of my most cherished honors came during my second year in academic medicine when I received the **Outstanding Clinical Instructor of the Year 1961-1962 Award,** given each year to a member of the faculty "In recognition of his outstanding ability to teach, interest in student welfare and devotion to the principles of medicine." The award came from the student body of the University of Louisville School of Medicine and the Student American Medical Association. This was remarkably gratifying at this early start into academic medicine. I attribute much of this success to experience in both private practice as well as research at Walter Reed and Ft. Detrick allowing me to promote scientifically-based medical practice. Whatever the reason, it seemed to stick because I received the **Award** again for **1963** and again in **1966-67.**

As I interacted with the Pediatric residents I realized there was an important body of knowledge that was being passed from generation to generation only by word of mouth and *in vivo* demonstrations. This included procedures for scalp vein infusions, bone marrow aspiration, cardiopulmonary resuscitation, exchange blood transfusions, insertion of urinary catheters, nasogastric intubation, etc. So, I wrote my first book with specific guides for state-of-the art techniques important to Pediatric practice.

The book **PEDIATRIC PROCEDURES** was published in 1964 by W. B. Saunders Co. (Philadelphia). Extensive illustration was required and my pretty little 3 yr. old daughter, Carla, served as a model for many of the drawings. The book was well received and soon translated and published in German and later in Spanish. Years later a second edition was published.

At the time I came to Louisville I was interested in directing my research to certain aspects of mycology such as the carcinogenic mycotoxins of *Aspergillus flavus*. At Ft. Detrick I learned of some fascinating aspects of fungi that needed further research. After presenting my proposed projects and the approaches to be taken to a Committee on Research Space I was given a new laboratory in the Medical Dental Research Building. I obtained some funding to provide a superb technician, Evelyn Shupp, and a scholarly post-doctoral fellow, **Sophia Franco, M.D.**, who had completed our residency program. I was given a brief sabbatical to go to the Mycology Laboratory at the Centers for Disease Control, USPHS, in Atlanta and complete a laboratory training program in diagnostic mycology. The productive output from our lab is shown in the Abstracts # 1 through 11, in **APPENDIX 2.**

A major component of the Department of Pediatrics was the modern four-story Children's Hospital **(FIG. 12-C)**, located directly across the street from the Louisville General Hospital. This was the third oldest Children's Hospital in the United States, founded in 1892 as Children's Free Hospital and originally located in a refurbished three-story townhouse at 220 E. Chestnut St. I mention here certain key factors in the origin of this historic children's' hospital in order to make comparisons later to the other children's' hospitals where I worked (St. Jude Children's Research Hospital, Le Bonheur Children's' Hospital and the Harriet Lane Home at the Johns Hopkins). Important to note today (2014) is the **absence** of governmental influence in the establishment of early hospitals and the delivery of competent healthcare; note the alternative resources.

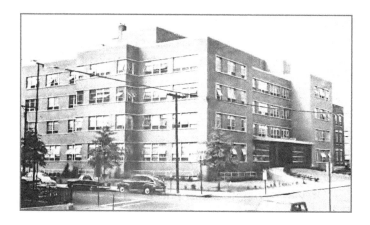

FIG. 12-C: Children's Hospital, 220 Chestnut, in the 1960s. Across street from Louisville General Hospital.

In the latter part of the 19th century, before the ***Flexner Report***, benevolent citizens of Louisville recognized the need for a facility exclusively for the treatment of children, often misfits in adult hospitals. Wisely, they realized more than building an edifice would be the need for operational support. I point out here, lest Jeanette and Carla complain, the essential leadership roles of **women** and the **church** in the establishment of the remarkable healthcare services for children that we enjoy today in the United States.

Local social activists Mary Lafon, Hallie Quigley and a small group of women from the Warren Memorial Presbyterian Church elicited the support of local physicians Dr. John A. Larrabee, president of the American Medical Association's Section on Children's Diseases and of the Louisville City Hospital College of Medicine and Dr. Ap Morgan, a pioneer in both surgery and orthopedics in the establishment of the **Children's Free Hospital.** Operation was to depend on volunteers and gifts, an extreme expression of faith. I ask you now – could this happen today? Nevertheless, a team of **volunteers** served as administrator (CEO), 99 percent of the working staff, public relations staff, and met monthly to sew large numbers of sheets, towels, diapers, etc. A newly formed Women's'

Club of Louisville also joined in to support the hospital. It is espe-
cially noteworthy that the **first 27 years of the operation** of the
Free Children's' Hospital was solely from altruistic efforts of these
Louisville volunteers.

The inclusion of several important scenes from Children's' Free
Hospital, in a book series by the famous Louisville author Annie
Fellows Johnston, entitled *"The Little Colonel's Holidays,"* (circa
1901, later made famous in Shirley Temple movies) enhanced national recognition. Contributions poured in from people giving
from what they had to help the children – flowers, Christmas trees,
Easter toys, clothing, coal, butter, apples, rabbits, sandwiches, wa-
termelons, apples, scrapbooks, seashells from Florida, etc. When
one has a noble and nonpolitical cause people respond voluntarily
without taxation. In 1910 a new building was erected and attached
to the house with an annex. **(FIG. 12-C)**

Dr. Alex Steigman was nationally recognized in the field of
Infectious Diseases as well as academic Pediatrics. I was not sur-
prised that he accepted an important position with the American
Academy of Pediatrics to head a new program for the training
of American pediatricians. Dr. Frank Falkner, an Americanized
Englishman and renowned in his own right in the field of Child
Growth and Development was appointed Chairman of the
Department.

By 1966, my fifth year at the University of Louisville, and now
36 years of age, I had been promoted to full Professor of Pediatrics
(1966); Assistant to the Chairman; Director of Pediatric Education;
Director of Infectious Diseases Unit; Chief of Pediatrics at Louisville
General Hospital (1963) and Consultant in Pediatrics to the U.S.
Army Ireland Hospital at Ft. Knox, Ky.

I have yet to understand why my career was being drawn in this
direction. I truly had no interest in being "chief of something" or in
faculty hierarchy; I preferred to work at the hands-on level following some laboratory research, clinical teaching and clinical trials.
Moreover, I was unable to understand the reasons for my academic
ladder advancement. Never in my life, then or later, did I ask to be

considered for promotion or a pay raise - it was just not a Hughes thing. Incidentally, promotions were more forthcoming than pay raises, perhaps a factor in easy promotions.

I was not a charismatic or brilliant personality, not a recipient of large grants and certainly not a prototype for leadership. I was one among many highly competent faculty members. I can only conclude that my difficulty in saying **No!** had drawn me away from a career I would prefer to pursue. My dear Jeanette's philosophy was precisely the same as mine. She was completely unimpressed by promotions, etc. and never encouraged me to take on more responsibilities. Her advice was often, **"Just say No!"** What would have been easy for her was difficult for me. Home with the family was her greatest goal. Now, at age 84 years I know she was right.

In the spring of 1965 Jeanette announced she was expecting a baby. This sent a shout of joy throughout the family tree. This time when we were asked the proverbial question, "Do you want a boy or a girl?" we could honestly say, "It doesn't matter." Before the birth of our third child we moved from our home in Moorgate to a real dream home on Cherokee Road on the edge of beautiful Cherokee Park near downtown Louisville. The stone Dutch Colonial classic with slate roof gave Jeanette ample imagination for a masterpiece of decor. On October 10, 1965 at 2:14 am in Methodist Evangelical Hospital our second son, **Christopher Blake Hughes**, was delivered by Dr. Peggy Howard, Jeanette's favorite Obstetrician. Dr. Richard Wolf, our friend and Pediatrician, told me our new son was healthy and assured me he would do well in life. He was correct. **(FIG.12-D)**.

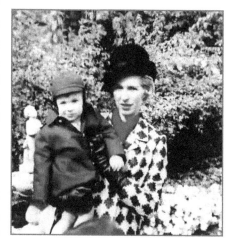

FIG. 12-D: Chris and Jeanette at home on Cherokee Road, Louisville, 1965.

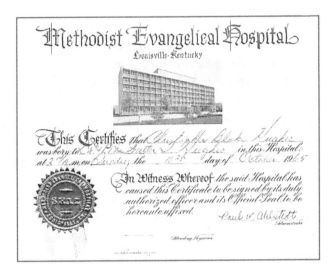

FIG. 12-E: Christopher Blake Hughes born on Oct. 10, 1965 in Louisville.

Another family blessing came from Louisville. My dear sister Katherine met a young man, John Thomas Moore, just out of graduate school in his first job as Comptroller of a restaurant chain. They had in common St. Paul Methodist Church and Tom's father was the beloved Director of Pharmacy at Children's Hospital. After their marriage Tom received his PhD. from the University of Kentucky and subsequently spent a career as a college professor, teaching business administration, first in Kentucky and later at Kennesaw College in Atlanta. Eventually, my mother, Katherine and her family and my brother Joe settled down for final years in Atlanta (only 110 miles from our home place in Cleveland, TN).

Space and time prevent me from commenting individually on each of my colleagues in the Department of Pediatrics at the University of Louisville so I am providing a cross-sectional listing of our department around the year of 1967, to chronicle their names in my mind and to acknowledge their services to the welfare of children.

FULL-TIME FACULTY:

Dr. Frank Falkner, M.D., M.R.C.P.
Professor and Chairman, Chief of Staff, Children's Hospital; and Associate in Psychiatry.

Dr. William Brodsky, M.D.
Professor of Research Pediatrics
Chief, Biophysical Chemistry

Dr. Walter Hughes, M.D.
Professor of Pediatrics; Assistant Chairman; Director of Pediatric Education; Chief of Pediatrics, Louisville General Hospital

Dr. Walton M. Edwards, M.D.
Associate Professor of Pediatrics; Chief of Pediatrics, Children's Hospital; Director House Staff Training; and Associate in Medicine

Dr. Kareem Minhaus, M.D.
Associate Professor of Pediatrics; Chief, Section of Pediatric Cardiology

Dr. Bernard Weisskopf, M.D.
Associate Professor of Pediatrics; Director, Child Evaluation Center

Dr. Ronald Wilson, PhD.
Associate Professor of Pediatrics, Child Psychology Research, CEC

Dr. Leonard Reisman, M.D.
Associate Professor of Pediatrics; Chief, Genetic Counseling Unit; Associate in Medicine, Pathology and Microbiology

Dr. Billy Andrews, M.D.	Associate Professor of Pediatrics, Director, High-Risk Infant Project, Associate in Microbiology, Obstetrics and Gynecology
Dr. Duncan MacMillian, M.D.	Assistant Professor of Pediatrics Director, Pediatric Endocrinology
Dr. Mary Smith, M.D.	Assistant Professor of Pediatrics, Director of Admissions, Children's' Hospital
Dr. Thomas Colley, PhD.	Assistant Professor of Pediatrics, Chief Psychologist, CEC
Dr. Carlos Gonzalez, M.D.	Assistant Professor of Pediatrics Section of Biophysical Chemistry
Dr. Theodore Schilb, PhD.	Instructor in Pediatrics Section Biophysical Chemistry
Dr. Adam Matheny PhD.	Assistant Professor of Pediatrics Neonatal Psychology
Dr. William Brown, PhD.	Assistant Professor of Pediatrics Director, Speech and Hearing
Dr. Bryan Hall, M.D.	Instructor in Pediatrics

ASSOCIATES IN PEDIATRICS:

Drs. S. Taha Anvari, MD (Neurology), Lawrence A. Davis, MD (Radiology), Charles W. Fishel, PhD (Microbiology), Helen M. Gray, MD (Psychiatry), Dominick Gentile MD (Renology), Paul Johnston, PhD (Microbiology), Giovannia Raccuglia MD (Hematology) and Donald Kmetz MD (Pathology).

VOLUNTARY FACULTY:

Professor Emeritus: Drs. Leonard Davidson, William Nicholson, and Harry Andrews.

Clinical Professors: Dr. Lee Palmer

Associate Clinical Professors: Drs. Martin Harris, John Larson, Margaret Limper, Owen Ogden, A.L. Roby, and Edwin Scott.

Assistant Clinical Professors: Drs. Billy Adams, Bernard Barron, Alvin Churney, Thomas Courtney, Kenneth Crawford, John Doyle, Louis Giesel, Richard Greathouse, Cathryn Handleman, Nathan Handleman, Kenneth Harris, Patrick Hess, Grace James, Martin Kaplan, Selby Love, Maurice Perellis, Elliot Podoll, Nan Robinson, Jo Ann Sexton, Clyde Sheldon, Louis Sternberg, Margaret Vermillion and Richard Wolf.

Clinical Instructors: Drs. Stiles Allen, Henry Delong, Nicholas Glazer, Arthur Issacs, Louis Kahle, John Karibo, Robert Kidd, Leslie Langley, Aaron Marcum, Geraldine Paxton, Carmine Scalzitti, Surjeet Singh and Glen Stout.

HOUSE STAFF:

Fellows: Drs. Francisco Elbl (Cardiology), Ronald N. Collier (Neonatology), Robert Howard (Comprehensive Pediatrics), Jerry Seligman (Neonatology).

Fifth Year Resident and Assistant Instructor: Dr. Chin Yong Chung.

Fourth Year Resident and Assistant Instructor: Dr. Nuhad Dinno.

Third Year Residents and Assistant Instructors: Drs. Leticia Chy-Koa, **Ho Kyun Kim** and Michael Nall.

Second Year Residents and Assistant Instructors: Drs. Chung-Ja Jung, Chong Bin Kim, Yung Hie Koh, Vichien Lorchirachookul, Faradj Masoudi, Iraj Rezvani, Neal Saunders and Victoria Yap.

First Year Residents and Assistant Instructors: Drs. **Sandor Feldman**, Robert Solinger, Vunne Thanapailal and Leticia Vizcarra.

Straight Intern in Pediatrics: Dr. Danny Strunk.

The Dann Byck Pediatric Residency: Dr. Keith Bachman, Dr. Bryan D. Hall and Dr. Kenneth Henderson.

I must mention here Dr. Richard Wan, who completed his residency before 1967 but who has stayed in continuous contact with me as a colleague and friend for more than 50 years.

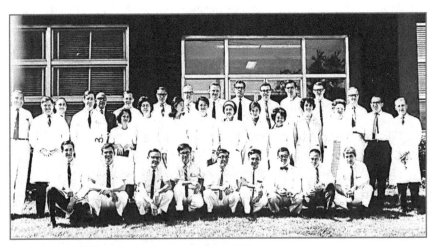

FIG. 12-F: THE HOUSE STAFF AND MEMBERS OF THE FULLTIME DEPARTMENT OF PEDIATRICS 1967.

While I was at Ft. Detrick I often attended Grand Rounds in Medicine on Saturday mornings at the Johns Hopkins Hospital in nearby Baltimore and met a young surgeon named Alex Haller, just finishing a fellowship there in Pediatric Surgery. A few days after I arrived in Louisville in 1961 I met Alex crossing the street from Louisville General Hospital to Children's Hospital. He had also just joined the faculty in the Department of Surgery. Right away Haller made a remarkable impact on Pediatric Surgery at Children's Hospital and LGH – a superb surgeon, fascinating speaker and teacher, dynamic personality and university citizen. We chatted fairly often in the coffee shop or in my office. Despite his exceptional productivity, his Chairman refused to designate him as Chief of Pediatric Surgery, a title clearly deserved – too young, he said. After a couple years or so passed he remained unrewarded and one day stopped in my office and told me he had just accepted an appointment as Chief of Pediatric Surgery at the Johns Hopkins University School of Medicine. As expected, Alex Haller became an icon in the field of Pediatric Surgery and spent the rest of his career at Hopkins. Serendipitously, years later I ended up at the same institution as Professor of Pediatrics and Director of the Division of Infectious Diseases with offices in the same building as Alex.

The faculty turnover in the Department of Pediatrics was not unusual for the relatively young productive group. Dr. William Brodsky and his research group moved to Mt. Siniai Medical School in New York. Dr. Leonard Reisman moved to Jefferson Medical College in Philadelphia. On balance, Dr. Billy Andrews was recruited as Director of Neonatology and contributed a lifetime of service and prestige to the University of Louisville and a lifetime of friendship to me. Billy had been a resident in Pediatrics at the Walter Reed Army Hospital while I was at the Walter Reed group at Ft. Detrick and at the time of Carla's birth at Walter Reed. However, I never really met him until he presented papers at the Southern Society for Pediatric Research in New Orleans. When I returned to Louisville I suggested to my Chairman, Frank Faulkner that he consider Billy for Director of Neonatology in our department. He did and Billy accepted.

I must mention one experience with Billy. His altruistic nature had led him early on to go beyond the academic gown and seek help for the newborn infants discharged from his nursery into inner city poverty. He asked me to join him as co-investigator in writing a grant to obtain funds for comprehensive services to high-risk infants and siblings in poor families. We reviewed reams of data from census tracts to establish a definition of "poverty" which was realistic. It was not until I was reading a final draft of the grant that I experienced a revelation. The next day I exclaimed to Billy, "I came from poverty!! Most of my early life was spent in poverty according to our criteria." This was truly the first time I ever thought of myself as being from a poor family. Well, I still don't feel poor. Nevertheless, the grant was funded for $640,000 per year for five years.

In 1967 Dr. Frank Falkner resigned as Chairman of the Department of Pediatrics to become Chief of the new Perinatal Biology and Infant Mortality Branch of the National Institute of Child Health and Human Development and Professor of Pediatrics at Georgetown University School of Medicine.

In late 1967 when the relatively new Dean of the Medical School, Donn L. Smith, MD, called me to his office **(Fig. 12-A)** I expected he would discuss an ad hoc committee to which he had assigned me to review student curriculum and faculty development. I had made a proposal in the committee to eliminate the traditional academic ranking of faculty (i.e. Assistant Professor, Associate Professor, Professor) because it had no functional purpose and consumed an inordinate amount of faculty time fiddling around in Promotions Committees and developing guidelines for promotion. Our committee had recently recommended the proposal and at a recent faculty meeting over 90% of the Faculty voted against it, not to our surprise.

Dean Smith had been a Colonel on General Patton's staff in World War II and had many attributes of Patton. The students presented him with pair of pearl-handled pistols for Christmas. He was making rather radical changes in the University of Louisville School of Medicine. I liked him, which made it difficult for me to respond to his proposal.

Coming directly to the point Dean Smith informed me that he had convened a Search Committee to find a new chairman for the Department of Pediatrics, that the committee had met and reviewed a list of candidates and had recommended the position be offered to me. He added he supported the recommendation and would like to enter into negotiations on the matter. There was no question in my mind, this was not something I wanted to do and if I did at 37 years of age it would set the direction for the rest of my career. Jeanette would have been proud of me when I just said **NO!** (politely, very politely). After a long discussion I agreed to serve as Acting Chairman of the Department of Pediatrics and Physician-in-Chief of Children's Hospital until a new Chairman could be found. At home Jeanette asked why they couldn't get someone else for Acting Chairman and predicted they would be coming back to me. A year later that was exactly the case, despite very good candidates like my close friend Dr. Billy Andrews.

By the end of 1968 I was at a career crossroad. I had received job offers from other institutions, but mostly for "Chairman" or "Chief" of something. Had I chosen this track I would stay in Louisville. Possibly by the Grace of God, I received a call from Dr. Donald Pinkel, Director of a new, almost unheard of St. Jude Children's Research Hospital in Jeanette's beloved Memphis, asking if I might be interested in coming to work exclusively in clinical and laboratory efforts in infectious diseases for the betterment of children with cancer.

After visits in 1968 to St. Jude Children's Research Hospital, founded in 1962, I resigned my job and accepted a position at St. Jude, along with an affiliated Professorship in Pediatrics at the University of Tennessee with my mentors James Ettledorf, James Hughes and others.

CHAPTER 13

St. Jude and Memphis – 1969 to 1977

"You're going where?" exclaimed an esteemed colleague and former mentor, now in Washington, when I told him I had declined the Chairmanship at the University of Louisville and was moving to Memphis.

"St. Jude Children's Research Hospital," I said again. "It's a new institution, opened only seven years ago to do research in childhood cancer and other catastrophic diseases of children," I answered.

"Never heard of it," he replied. "Why are you thwarting a very promising career in academia? I expected someday you might move on to a more prestigious job, but this is not it. What led you to this decision - and a cancer hospital?"

I don't recall the details of my lengthy explanation but I do recall it was not convincing. Now, as I am trying to recall my story for this chapter and to tell my grandchildren why I left a good job, a beautiful place to live, and close friends, to move to a strikingly different place, I am still having trouble putting forth a convincing argument.

In retrospect, some half a century later, I can look more objectively at the factors involved. I had earlier adequately stated my reasons for preferring a career in hands-on clinical and laboratory research rather than climbing the traditional academic ladder to

Professor, Chairman, Dean, National Societies, etc. I had concluded I could not, or would not do both. That was understandable to most of my colleagues. What I have trouble with even now is to tell you why I came to St. Jude over other options.

Firstly, what advantages did St. Jude offer over our Department of Pediatrics in Louisville, a measure I applied to all the options I considered? If compared by size our Children's Hospital **(FIG. 12-C)** alone was more than double the size of the St. Jude institution **(FIG. 13-A)**, not to mention wards, nursery, clinics and offices at Louisville General Hospital **(FIG. 12-B)**, research laboratories in the new Medical-Dental Research Building and some satellite projects. By now I had a large corner office with windows on the top floor of Children's Hospital, compared to a 9 x 12er next to X-ray room at St. Jude. Laboratory space for me would potentially be greater than my lab in Louisville. Salaries were similar; rank was similar Professor/ Member and I would be designated as Chief of the Infectious Diseases Service (IDS) at St. Jude. While I would be the only person in IDS, I would have the option to build a group if it could be justified by productivity or to just work alone.

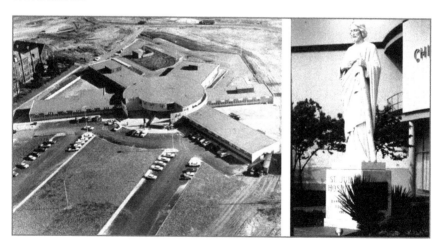

FIG. 13-A: St. Jude Children's Research Hospital when I arrived in 1969.

The Department of Pediatrics in Louisville had the faculty listed in Chapter 12 and St. Jude had the following full-time Faculty in 1968: Donald Pinkel, MD (Medical Director); H. Omar Hustu, MD (Radiology); Warren Johnson, MD (Pathology); Luis Borella, MD (Immunology and Hematology); David Kingsbury, MD (Virology); Thomas Walters,MD (Hematology); Paulus Zee, MD, PhD (Nutrition and Metabolism); Jose Burdman, MD (Pharmacology); Charles Pratt, MD (Chemotherapy); Charlene Holton, MD(Oncology); Joe Simone, MD (Hematology); John W. Smith, MD (Virology); Alben Curtis, DMD (Dentistry); Herbert Ennis, PhD (Pharmacology); Allan Granoff, PhD (Virology); Martin Morrison, PhD (Biochemistry); Bruce Sells, PhD (Biochemistry); Thomas Avery, PhD (Animal Science); R.W. Darlington, PhD (Virology); Leon Journey, PhD (Pharmacology); DeWayne Roberts, PhD (Pharmacology); Robert Webster, PhD (Immunology); Wai Yiu Cheung, PhD (Biochemistry); Maneth Gravell, PhD (Virology); William Groves, PhD (Biochemistry); Ahmed Halbeeb, PhD (Immunology); and Lois Kucera, PhD (Virology).

I point out that all of these faculty members were the pioneering first generation of St. Jude researchers and all had been there less than seven years. None had reached professional celebrity status and all had been recruited for research in childhood cancer. Furthermore, all of the 27 full-time faculty, including the Medical Director, were less than 45 years of age (Pinkel was 34 yr. old when he became Director in 1962). None of the faculty had a research interest in the field of Infectious Diseases. The Virologists were basic scientists interested in the role of viruses as a cause of cancer, with the exception of Rob Webster, PhD, who was focused on the antigenic structure of *avian influenza* viruses, totally unrelated to what I would do.

The recruitment of an Infectious Diseases "Specialist" to St. Jude arose out of necessity more than a strategic design for a major research program. The necessity was due to the fact that fatal infectious diseases were interfering with the success of the newly developed "Total Therapy" regimens that were providing cures for acute lymphocytic leukemia. Most of these infections were not those commonly seen in children, but rather the so-called "Opportunistic Infections" that were emerging in the 1960s in immunocompromised hosts with cancer, congenital immunodeficiency disorders, and organ transplant recipients. Unfortunately, a body of knowledge and experts to deal with these unfamiliar infections such as systemic candidiasis, aspergillosis, disseminated cytomegalovirus disease, *Pneumocystis carinii* pneumonia, *Pseudomonas* sepsis, etc. were woefully lacking. Although I had some basic research experiences at Ft. Detrick, had established a research laboratory in Mycology in Louisville and had a few publications of "odd" infections, I was no expert in the problems occurring at St. Jude. However, I had realized earlier that the area of infectious diseases I wished to pursue was that of the immunocompromised host. Unless new methods were developed to prevent, diagnose and treat these opportunistic infections, progress in many fields of Medicine would be impeded.

Another issue I faced was that one of the other job offers I was considering was in the Department of Pediatrics at the University of Tennessee College of Medicine and Le Bonheur Children's Hospital also in Memphis. Dr. James G. Hughes, Chairman, had invited me for a recruitment visit earlier to join his department and establish a new Division of Pediatric Infectious Diseases. The position had been offered to me as well as the faculty appointment of Professor of Pediatrics. I felt honored by this confidence and the opportunity to work again with Dr. Ettledorf along with other esteemed colleagues. The two positions were very different; UT was the traditional academic world and St. Jude was unexplored territory. Choosing either would lead to hard feelings from the other. Of the UT group perhaps only Dr. Ettledorf appreciated why I chose St. Jude although Dr. Hughes provided me a faculty appointment as Professor of Pediatrics because the entire St. Jude faculty received UT faculty status without pay.

As I re-read the paragraphs above, I realize I have in no way answered the question, "Why did you choose St. Jude?" I can do that now with complete clarity in my own mind. The answer is, **The Interview,** it was the reason.

For my first interview at St. Jude I arrived in Memphis on a Thursday afternoon. Dr. Don Pinkel, Medical Director of St. Jude, met me at the airport arrival gate and drove me directly to St. Jude in his ten-year old station wagon, cluttered with children's school debris and dust. Already the interview was different from others I had done where I had been instructed to take a cab to a nice hotel and where someone would meet me for dinner at a plush restaurant.

Pinkel and I arrived around 4:00 pm at St. Jude, located at a downtown site I had never seen during my years in Memphis because it was in a slum/poverty area of the city. As we reached the entrance to the new two-story, star-shaped building **(FIG.13-A)**, an elderly smiling African-American security guard opened the door but not before Pinkel introduced us, Mr. Willis was his name. Once inside, we began a tour of the facilities, which took a couple of hours due to explanations of not only what was happening at each site, but also what was needed and what was planned.

After another hour of talk about St. Jude in his small office, he mentioned we were going to have dinner at his home and his wife was expecting us by 7:30 pm to grill steaks and hot dogs in the backyard with his family. His modest home reflected a busy family life with his nine children. I believe seven children were home at the time and his wife, Marita, made me feel welcome and comfortable. After dinner we talked more about St. Jude and I felt free to express my opinion on what I believed important for the health and welfare of children. He delivered me to a nearby Holiday Inn Motel near midnight and informed me he would pick me up in the morning – at about 7:00 am. So far, the interview visit had been unconventional to say the least.

At breakfast in the hospital cafeteria Don pointed out that this was the institutional dining room that everyone used, doctors, patients, parents, and all employees. He knew the first name of every employee from housekeepers to doctors and spoke to them in passing.

"Some of the faculty wanted a separate dining room because

they felt uncomfortable seeing some of the sick patients in wheel chairs with IVs and hair loss," Pinkel said. "So, I told them no, they needed to feel uncomfortable and what they found offensive was why they were here."

A large table in the middle of the cafeteria was filled with baskets of apples, oranges, and bananas and a galvanized tub with small cartons of milk on ice. "We keep the table stocked at all times so children and parents can come by and take what they want for free. In fact parents take all their meals here for free. We have no vending machines at St. Jude because we promote good nutrition and 'cokes' are not good nutrition."

The clocks throughout the building were 24-hour clocks, reminding me of my army days. "We believe it's the best way to designate time and it helps avoid confusion with AM and PM. We are totally on the metric system for the same reason. Also, we use generic names for drugs and do not use brand names. In fact the pharmaceutical company representative must apply through our Pharmacy office to meet with any of our physicians. Our Chief of Pharmacy, Larry Barker, is into these new computer systems and we are in the process of making the Pharmacy a data hub for clinical uses."

"I don't recall seeing the business offices," I said to Don as we walked to my first appointment at 8:30 AM.

"We don't have one. There are no charges of any kind to our patients. Even if they are able to pay we don't allow them to do so.

"A stipulation of our founder, Danny Thomas, was that all patients, regardless of race, creed, religion and socio-economic status be afforded the services of St. Jude at no cost – in a sense a Free Children's Hospital. This came from a religious experience while he was a struggling unknown entertainer in Chicago. Despondent and forlorn he prayed to St. Jude Thaddeus, patron saint of hopeless causes, 'Show me my way in life and I will build you a shrine'. A remarkable success followed and when famous and wealthy he came to make good his promise. He sought the advice of Cardinal Samuel Stritch, the Catholic Archbishop of Chicago who suggested the shrine be a free hospital for children and that it be located in Memphis. Fortunately, he followed the advice of Dr. Lemuel Diggs, a research hematologist and Professor of Medicine at the University of Tennessee College of Medicine and involved in Thomas' early visits and plans. Diggs suggested he build a research center for incurable childhood diseases rather than a free hospital because even the federal government could not afford that and pointed out that Memphis already had Le Bonheur Children's Hospital and Frank T. Tobey Children's Hospital that provided the needed services for children in Memphis. Of course, that's what he did but insisting on no charges for any patient or parent."

Later we continued a discussion of financial matters. The basis of St. Jude's financing was volunteers. I was reminded of the Free Children's Hospital in Louisville, founded and operated for 27 years by volunteers and women of the church. Danny had wisely recruited the aid of an established group of volunteer fundraisers namely the American Lebanese Syrian Associated Charities (ALSAC). These were Americans, like Danny, of Middle East descent who had banded together in chapters across the U. S. to raise funds for various charity projects within their communities in appreciation for the opportunities they had experienced in America. Now, they were directing all their efforts to the funding of St. Jude. In 1968 ALSAC had raised $1,321,098.47 for the annual St. Jude budget. Impressed as I was, I could never have imagined that in 2014-5, the time of this writing, that the projected fund raising from ALSAC alone would be one billion dollars for the year.

I digress a moment to comment on the role churches and religion have played in the establishment of hospitals and care of the suffering sick. I only need to mention names to make the point: **St. Jude** Children's' Research Hospital, **St. Christopher's** Children's' Hospital, **St. Joseph's** Hospital, **St. Frances** Hospital, **Baptist** Hospital, **Methodist** Hospital, **St. Mary's** Hospital, **Jewish** Hospital, **St. Luke-Presbyterian** Hospital, **Lutheran** Hospital, etc.

Pinkel's plan for St. Jude was to develop an institution focused on the health and welfare of children through research. The faculty would be equally divided with one-half as physician-scientists (MD) and one-half as basic scientists (PhD) mixed together under one roof provided with the opportunities to pursue promising research goals without the burden of writing grants and pressure to publish in order to survive. The measure of success would be productive research, clinical or basic science that would impact the prevention and cure of diseases of childhood. He pointed out that he wanted his researchers to focus on the **big picture**. "We started with the goal to **cure** leukemia, not to better understand the disease, not to search for causes, not to get NIH grants or even to develop new drugs; rather we went for the **cure** by any way we could get there."

My role would be to deal with the problems of infectious diseases in children with cancer. He foresaw infection as a limiting factor in further development of immunosuppressive chemotherapy for cancer as well as the developing area of organ transplantation. He needed someone to help the oncologists in dealing with current problems; and, he realized the body of knowledge and expertise for these infection problems were lacking. I would have the freedom to develop a research effort in any way I saw fit and he would provide the support needed – provided it was of scientific and applied merit.

I recall that I met Joe Simone, Charles Pratt, Paulus Zee and Rob Webster and memory fails to recall the others. I was impressed with the zest and zeal of these new St. Jude recruits and that I was in line with their ambitions for work at St. Jude.

So, what did I decide and why? Back home Jeanette said, "It would be nice to be back in Memphis near my mother and dad, but you decide what is best for you." I had also thought about what would be best for Jeanette and my children and concluded their opportunities in Memphis would be about the same as those in Louisville, possibly even better. The **interview** at St. Jude and talk with **Jeanette** left me with an unequivocal decision to move to Memphis. So, we did. You can conclude why.

In Memphis we were fortunate to find a charming old English Tudor house in Hein Park adjacent the campus of Rhodes College (formerly Southwestern University) and across the street (North Parkway) from the large midtown Overton Park where Jeanette and I had our first date (chapter 9). About three miles down N. Parkway was St. Jude Children's Research Hospital. Along the way was Snowden Elementary School where our children would attend, Evergreen Presbyterian Church where we sinfully changed from Methodists to Presbyterians and Rhodes College (Southwestern) School of Music where Carla could continue piano lessons. Schools, park and church were in walking distance and I could ride my bike to St. Jude if I wished to do so. Perfect main street America!

After a few days at work I seemed to know every employee by name and job. Mrs. Hazel Moody was the secretary assigned to me and had a tiny ante-office adjacent to mine. A gracious senior southern lady with executive demeanor and typing skills, she was my encyclopedia for St. Jude and was one of those remarkable people who knew how to get things done. At this time the latest in word processing was an electric Royal typewriter, carbon paper and the new innovation of liquid White-out. Photocopiers and cell phones were yet to come. An empty lab on the same floor but near the Clinical Laboratories had been assigned to me. I would recruit a technician.

I had no budget as such. Don Pinkel said most of the faculty didn't have a budget. "If you need supplies and equipment just call Clyde Davidson in Purchasing and tell him what you need. He has the supplier's catalogues and will get it for you. If you need to add people, we'll discuss it and then the Personnel office will find some candidates for you to interview. I don't think our faculty should be burdened with paper work and budgets. They are here to do research."

I immediately realized, more than expected, the serious threat infectious diseases was imposing on these children with cancer as well as the potential impact on the curative advances underway at St. Jude. At the same time I could see, more than I had expected, that much could be done to reduce the infectious burden using standard principles of infection control. The Clinical Laboratories were state-of-the-art for hematological, immunological and bio-chemical procedures, but microbiology was almost nonexistent. One med tech was responsible for bacteriology and Gram stains, in addition to doing blood counts and urinalysis in her spare time. I recall she cried a lot because the doctors were coming to her to tell them what was causing infection in their patients and she could not help. One of the nurses was responsible for reporting hospital-acquired infections. Visiting policies were liberal because of the critical nature of children with cancer. I had no data on infection rates, nosocomial or community acquired, for St. Jude. Fortunately, the individual patient medical record was superb.

Wisely, Pinkel had invested heavily in a system of medical re-cords. Expanding into several volumes a patient's record was the source of all information related to that patient. In addition to that of traditional hospital records it included all research protocol data, copies of protocols, photographs at time of admission and at subsequent intervals and lesions, detailed pathology reports and more. Daily progress notes were detailed by the physician. An index system by the medical records librarians coded medical episodes. The Chief of Medical Records was feared by all because she was relentless in demanding accuracy and completeness of entries from everyone from Pinkel to the newest nurse. I mention the medical record because it provided me a major tool with which to plan my strategy for an Infectious Diseases program at St. Jude.

From day one I had calls from the Hematology/Oncology doc-tors for consultations on their patients with fever and infection problems. By the end of the first month I decided to make rounds on all patients on the inpatient service each morning and to meet and take part daily with Dr. Joe Simone and his staff rounds held in the ward conference room at 10 am (including Saturday} when every hospitalized patient was reviewed and decisions on manage-ment made.

Because I was the only Pediatric Infectious Diseases special-ist in Memphis, had come through the UT-Le Bonheur system and held an appointment of Professor of Pediatrics I soon began to be deluged with calls from Pediatricians in private practice and at Le Bonheur Children's Hospital to see their patients in consultation. The most painful event of my new job was to say "No" to my colleagues and to limit my extra St. Jude work to scheduled teaching rounds and conferences in the Dept. of Pediatrics at Le Bonheur and Frank T. Tobey Hospitals.

During my first year and for some time thereafter, I made rounds alone on all patients every day, 7 days a week, seeing any patient with signs of infection or at risk for infection, whether or not requested. Most of the chemotherapy was administered in the outpatient clinic so the inpatients were there because of complications – usually fever and neutropenia and various infections. I put my notes in the chart for the attending oncologist to see. I could help with some patients, but for others I had little to offer. My aim was to see as many patients as possible to learn about their diseases. I had no interns, residents, students or fellows, so I had a rare privilege for academic professors of my day to be totally alone with the patient, one-on-one. I reviewed all x-rays of my patients with the radiologist, located two rooms down the hall from my office and attended the autopsy of all who died. The autopsy rate was 85 % of deaths and the awesome pathologist, Dr. Warren Johnson personally performed all autopsies followed by a clinical-pathological conference. This is how I learned about infections in the immuno-suppressed host. I could do this because of freedom from administrative responsibilities, cooperative colleagues, lack of bureaucracy of committees, grant writing, etc. and a keen desire to learn more.

I spent weeks in the medical records office collecting data to determine prevalence and incidence of specific infections and detailed analysis of well-documented cases. Nothing was computerized so I tabulated data by hand on large two-foot wide data forms.

I soon came to focus on the problems of *Pneumocystis carinii* pneumonia because of its increasing prevalence, burden on the institution and affect on patients who were being cured of leukemia (see chapter 14). The value of data from records review is evident from FIG.14-B.

I visited some other cancer centers to learn their approaches to the infection problem. At M. D. Anderson Cancer Center in Houston, **Dr. Gerald Bodey,** a Hematology/Oncology Internist was actively pursuing methods to deal with infections in cancer patients and had established some "germ-free" isolator units to protect susceptible infections. He was very helpful to me and became a lifetime friend and colleague and an icon in the field of infections in the immunocompromised host. He visited St Jude at my request. Similarly, **Dr. Stephen Schimpff** at the University of Maryland Cancer Center provided important information along with years of support. He later became Dean of the University Of Maryland. A third center I visited was the cancer unit at the Clinical Center at the National Institutes of Health in Bethesda where a young Pediatric Hematology/Oncology physician, **Phillip Pizzo, M.D**. was beginning to focus his attention to the problem of infections and had worked with a "Life Island Isolator" unit for severely immunodeficient children. He too became a lifetime colleague, a leader in the field and ended up as Dean at Stanford University. Unfortunately for my quest, little if any experience and knowledge of *Pneumocystis carinii* pneumonia was found.

Dr. Myron Schultz, Director of the Parasitic Disease Drug Department at the Centers for Disease Control (CDC), allowed me to spend time in his office to review case reports of *Pneumocystis carinii* submitted to the CDC for pentamidine therapy. At the end of my visits I became more convinced of the opportunity we had at St. Jude to advance the field.

Because of its importance to both St. Jude and me I have devoted a separate chapter (Chapter 14) to *Pneumocystis carinii* pneumonia during my early days at St. Jude and Chapter 17 to later contributions.

By the end of my first year or so we had instituted strict well-defined Infection Control Policies for the clinic and hospital; installed one "Isolator" unit in one room; added hand-wash stations; removed live-in activities for parents; re-constituted an Infection Control Committee; arranged an administrative assistant (**Mr. Land**

and later **Bobby Williams**) to manage compliance to infection control policies; added a clinical diagnostic laboratory in Mycology which I ran; established guidelines for the empiric treatment of patients with fever and neutropenia with intensive antibiotic therapy as proposed by Schimpff and later by Pizzo.

I learned right away no one likes strict infection control policies and heard complaints regularly from parents, nurses and some doctors. I recall telling Don Pinkel about a report I had read in the journal *Lancet* that vases of cut flowers in hospitals were a source of heavy *Pseudomonas aeruginosa* growth and that I thought because we were seeing such infections we should remove all vases of cut flowers from our patient-care areas. Whereupon Don picked up his phone, called the Head of Housekeeping and told them to remove all cut flowers and that in the future none would be allowed in the hospital. So, it was done before dark on the same day. The next day Mrs. Moody handed me a handful of messages from relatives, parents, nurses, and local florists about – you know what. Eventually, the president of the America Florist Association called; I referred the call to Mr. Land. Pinkel provided unrelenting support for infection control policies.

After a year or so I began to acquire people in addition to Mrs. Moody and Candace Miller, my research technician. I had requests for a Fellowship in Infectious Diseases from two of my former Pediatric Residents at the University of Louisville, **Dr. Sandor Feldman** and **Dr. Ho Kyun Kim**. They were the first Infectious Diseases Fellows at St. Jude and they did us proud. I first came to know Sandy Feldman as a junior medical student at the University of Louisville and was pleased to have him as a Fellow. He spent much of his subsequent career at St. Jude with stellar contributions to clinical research and ended up as head of Pediatric Infectious Diseases and the Billy Guyton Professor at the University of Mississippi (see chapter 14). Dr. Ho Kim made an important contribution by showing *Pneumocystis carinii* in humans to differ from that in the rat **(APPENDIX 1)**. Also, in 1970 **Dr. John W. Smith,** an Assistant Member of the faculty who had completed a Hem/

Oncology Fellowship at St. Jude became interested in *Pneumocystis carinii* and requested to transfer from Virology-Immunology to the Infectious Diseases Service to pursue some laboratory studies. He did and was successful in showing the chitin component of the cyst wall of the organism and suggested it was a fungus rather than a protozoan **(APPENDIX 1 and 2).**

Because most of the inpatients were hospitalized due to infection and we had asked for the addition of a Contagious Isolation Unit and a room to be designated Intensive Care Unit to manage patients with septic shock and *P. carinii* pneumonia; and because the largest part of the clinical operation for cancer therapy was in the outpatient department, Dr. Pinkel asked me to be Chief of the Inpatient component of the hospital and Dr. Joe Simone to be in Chief of the Outpatient department which we agreed to do. (Jeanette said, "Why couldn't someone else do that?")

Because we had no area for effective isolation of highly contagious infections such as chickenpox, a known fatal hazard to cancer patients, I obtained on loan an old Mobile Clinic Trailer used in earlier days for Tuberculosis Screening from the Memphis and Shelby County Health Department and parked it near the back door of the 27- room Inpatient Department. The St. Jude Maintenance Department under the direction of Mr. John Johnson adapted it for use and this provided a much-needed site to hold patients who might be highly infectious. Also, **Dr. Lorin Angier,** a Pediatric Cardiologist from the UT Dept. of Pediatrics was hired to serve as cardiologist at St. Jude, to aid in the intensive care of patients and to study left ventricular function in septic shock and was administratively in the Infectious Diseases Service by the end of 1970.

The rapid growth of St. Jude was exceeding the capacity of the original star-shaped, two-story physical facility opened in 1962.

In early 1971 Don Pinkel announced plans for the construction of a six-story, 90,000 sq. ft. addition to St. Jude for new and additional inpatient units, research labs and auditorium. I received a hand-written memo from Don. I had previously noticed that big requests from him came in a memo rather than the usual phone call and that the magnitude of the request was inversely proportional to the size of his cursive writing. This note was really tiny. He asked if I would "draw up some plans for a two-floor state-of-the-art inpatient hospital," stating Joe was dealing with a new outpatient area and Rob Webster would suggest plans for basic science research labs. These would be submitted to the architect.

I spent many months researching literature, consulting with engineers of various fields, visiting other institutions, reviewing the old Ft. Detrick containment facilities, and creative contemplation. Especially helpful was the critical review of my plans by Dr. Philip Brachman, Chief of the Epidemiology Program at the Centers of Diseases Control and his staff (George Mallison, Chief of Microbiological Control; Richard Kaslow, Hospital Epidemiologist; Wallace Rhodes, Mechanical Engineer; and Julia Garner, Hospital Infection Control). The design was strikingly radical and different from any other hospital, old or new. Later I learned the architects had told Don that we did not need to provide them our plans that that was their job. Pinkel's response was, "No! **We** tell **you** what we want and your job is to build it." And it was so.

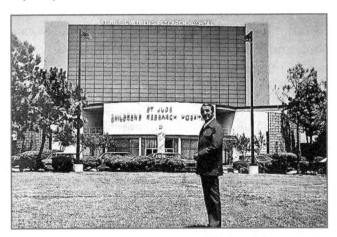

FIG. 13-B: New Six-story addition to St. Jude Children's Research Hospital opened in 1975.
Danny Thomas in foreground. Photo by Don Lancaster.

In June, 1975 the new inpatient facility on the 5th and 6th floors of the new building opened with each room under unidirectional air flow and 6 to 8 air exchanges per hour of outside air **(FIG. 13-B)**. All air entering rooms was filtered through 95% DOP high-efficiency filters and 30 %- efficiency prefilters, with no recirculated air. Pressure gradients for airflow at entrances existed in both protective and contagious isolation rooms. Each patient room had a parent and visitor room separated by a glass wall where anyone, parents, friends and pets, could come at any time without any risk to the patient. A four-bed Intensive Care Unit was developed with continuous negative pressure chambers used in the management of patients with *P. carinii* pneumonia, and designed by **Dr. S. K. Sanyal**, a cardiologist, who had replaced Dr. Angier (see chapter 14). An inner nursing and service area provided immediate access to nurses and other staff. The new St. Jude design gained national recognition and provided unique safety measures for our patients.

Of the some 27 full-time faculty at St. Jude when I arrived, I was the only Tennessean; others were predominantly from "up north." So, all of the faculty wives were in foreign territory and banded together as "The St. Jude Wives' Club." They met socially to comfort each other and to volunteer their services to St. Jude. Jeanette was also the first Tennessean in The Club and added the flavor of a southern lady to the group along with that of Sarah Pratt from Virginia. Jeanette's favorite role was to serve at the cake parties for St. Jude patients. In addition to birthdays, cake parties were held for each patient who successfully completed their chemotherapy in remission, usually meaning cure of their cancer. At home she was busy with three young children in school, restoration of our English Tudor house, coffee with neighbors, visiting relatives and always being there for me.

Racial turmoil was silently affecting our lives, especially after the assassination of Dr. Martin Luther King in 1968 some 5 miles from our house. "White flight" to the suburbs left mid-town and downtown vacancies among businesses and residencies. Our beloved First Methodist Church was left with an elderly membership and limited programs for our children, so we moved our church membership to the nearby Evergreen Presbyterian Church on the campus of the Presbyterian-founded Rhodes College, an excellent program at this time. Busing of Memphis students was evolving, despite any solid data to support effectiveness in education improvement for African-Americans.

Snowden School was 80 % White and 20 % Black because of compatible adjoining neighborhoods of middle-class White and Black professionals. To equalize the ratio, busing of White students out and Black students in was required, greatly stressing the City budget and putting Memphis children on buses early in the mornings to travel back and forth across Memphis to distant schools. This disrupted our Snowden School with which Jeanette and I had been so pleased.

Before the busing I recall one of our young sons had a Black classmate friend, named Tommy, I believe. One weekend Tommy came to our house to play. Later our son went to Tommy's house to play and on return Jeanette asked about his visit. "We had fun," he said, "and guess what Mom, Tommy's Mom is Black." I remember this vividly today because I thought this is the way it should be – young children look at each other and play together without thinking of race. One of my regrets in life is my failure to stand up and more vigorously oppose the busing movement which I had no doubt was wrong for both White and Black but I failed to become effectively involved. Opposition was "politically incorrect" within my social group, including St. Jude. So, I reluctantly went along with the crowd. It was all wrong!

Now, back to work. I realize that most of you are not interested in the nitty-gritty details of my workdays at St. Jude, so I'll spare you, as I tried to do with Jeanette and the children. Nevertheless, a few may be curious so I have added my standard **Curriculum vitae** in **APPENDIX 2** and written separate chapters (Chapters 14 and 17) on *Pneumocystis* pneumonia which represents a major part of my research at St. Jude. In addition, the following is a summary of the most significant research from our Infectious Diseases group up through 1977. Note the co-investigators in parenthesis and see references and abstracts in **APPENDIX 2** for more details. I always included the names of our essential **Research nurses** as co-investigators in clinical studies and wish to acknowledge their work again here.

1971:

- First study to show that *P. carinii* pneumonitis can recur after successful treatment and recovery (Hughes, Johnson).

1972:

- First report of the use of varicella zoster immune globulin (VZIG) in the immunosuppressed host exposed to varicella (Brunell, Gershon, Hughes).

- Antibacterial effects of methotrexate, *in vivo* and *in vitro* (Metcalf, Hughes).

1973:

- First study of thermophilic mycoflora in man and environment (Hughes, Crosier).

- First study of intravenous alimentation in children with cancer (Summers, Zee, Hughes).

1974:

- First study of disseminated histoplasmosis in children with cancer (Cox, Hughes).

- Efficiency of trimethoprim-sulfamethoxazole (TMP-SMZ) in the prevention and treatment of *P. carinii* pneumonia (Hughes, McNabb, Makres). **See Chapter 14.**

- Demonstration that protein-calorie malnutrition provokes *P. carinii* pneumonitis in both rats and humans (Hughes, Price, Sisko)

- First study of continuous negative pressure system for assisted ventilation in severe pneumonia (Sanyal, MacGraw, Hughes).

1975:

- First study to delineate the clinical features and outcome of varicella in cancer patients (Feldman, Hughes, Daniel).

1976:

- Report of first case of Kawasaki's disease in continental United States (Brown, Billmeier, Cox).

- Identification of cyclic 3', 5'-nucleotide phosphodiesterase of *Candida albicans* (Gunasesekaren, Hughes, Pearson).

1977:

- First report of *P. carinii* in gastric contents and use of aspirate for diagnosis of *P. carinii* pneumonitis (Chan, Pifer, Hughes).

- Successful use of chemoprophylaxis for *P. carinii* pneumonitis in cancer patients (Hughes, Kuhn, Chaudhary). **Chapter 14.**

- First scanning electron microscopic studies of *P. carinii* (Murphy, Pifer, Hughes).

- First *in vitro* propagation of *P. carinii* (Pifer, Hughes, Murphy).

To provide a comprehensive perspective of my experience with **Pneumocystis carinii** pneumonia I have devoted two chapters (14 and 17) to this topic and to justify "Pneumocystis" in the title of my memoir.

Pneumocystis Pneumonia: Early Years at St. Jude, 1969-1977

I expect some of you may not be familiar with *Pneumocystis* so I'll give a brief background of the organism and the disease it causes and then focus on the menace it created in the early days of St. Jude Children's Hospital, tell how we dealt with it and how the St. Jude solutions have been applied to contemporary circumstances. What follows here and in Chapter 17 is included in the **Danny Thomas Series Lecture** (available on CD) I was privileged to deliver during the **50th Anniversary Celebration** at St. Jude in 2012.

Background

In 1909 the famous Brazilian parasitologist Carlos Chagas reported his findings of heretofore unrecognized stages in the life cycle of the protozoan *Trypanosma cruzi* in rats. A year after Chagas' paper was published Dr. Antonio Carini, an Italian microbiologist at the Pasteur Institute in Sao Paulo, Brazil reported similar findings in rats infected with *Trypanosoma lewisi*. He also concluded that these were stages in the life cycle of trypanosomes. The clincher came in 1912 when the Delanoes, a husband-wife team at the Pasteur Institute in Paris, published a three-page article describing the cyst forms in the lungs of rats not infected with trypanosomes. They showed convincingly that the cysts of Chagas and Carini were a new organism and suggested the name *Pneumocystis* because the cysts were found only in the lung and *carinii* because Dr. Carini had provided specimens for their study. Later Chagas and Carini agreed on these findings.

For the next 30 years little attention was given to the organism except for reports of *P. carinii* in rats, guinea pigs, rabbits and monkeys in Brazil, rats and mice in England and rats in Switzerland.

During the 1940s and World War II epidemics of a mysterious interstitial plasma cell pneumonitis of unknown etiology killed thousands of infants in Europe. Two Dutch workers, van der Meer and Brugge in 1942 were the first to show the cause to be *P. carinii.* This was the first report of the infection in humans.

With economic recovery and reconstruction after World War II the epidemics subsided.

During the 1950s sporadic cases of *Pneumocystis carinii* pneumonia (PCP) began to appear but more in children and adults with congenital immunodeficiency and cancer than in infants. The first case in the United States was reported in 1954.

As more cases were reported in the U. S., The Centers for Disease Control (CDC) obtained a supply of the drug pentamidine isethionate from England, the only drug known to have activity against PCP. The drug was highly toxic and not approved by the FDA. It was made available on a case-by-case basis to physicians for use in documented cases.

In 1969 Dr. Myron Shultz, Director of the Parasitic Disease Drug Branch of the CDC noticed that an excessive number of requests for pentamidine were coming from St. Jude Children's Research Hospital in Memphis – the smallest hospital of them all. So, an on-site CDC investigation was ordered. After several weeks of searching the investigation was reported in the **Journal of the American Medical Association.**

Pneumocystis carinii
Pneumonia in a Hospital
for Children   JAMA, Nov 9, 1970

From the Parasitic Diseases Branch,
Epidemiology Program, National Com-
municable Disease Center

Epidemiologic Aspects

David R. Perera, MD; Karl A. Western, MD; H. Durell Johnson, MD;
Warren W. Johnson, MD; Myron G. Schultz, DVM, MD, DCMT; and Philip V. Akers, MA

The first large outbreak of Pneumocystis carinii *pneumonia
reported in the United States occurred at St. Jude Children's Research Hospital in Memphis.*

**FIG. 14-A: Report of epidemic at St. Jude Children's Research
Hospital in 1970.**

This was not the publicity a new hospital less than seven years
old needed. The investigation found that 19 documented cases
of PCP had occurred from the time the hospital opened in 1962
and the CDC visit in 1969. Importantly, 17 of the cases had occurred in the last two years from 1967 through 1969. The cause
was deemed to be due to more intensive immunosuppressive
therapy in recent years required to achieve greater survival rates
and cure from malignancies, rather than any source of infection
or contagion pattern.

I came to St. Jude as Chairman of the Department of Infectious
Diseases soon after the CDC dudes left. Actually, it wasn't a department at the time and was referred to as the Infectious Diseases
Service. My Chairmanship was near ideal with no one in the department, no committee meetings, no requests for pay raise or
promotions, adequate budget provided, and, grant writing as op-
tional. It was my very best year as a departmental chairman. I'm

now convinced The Director, Dr. Donald Pinkel, had devised these faculty benefits as a ploy leaving me nothing to do but research.

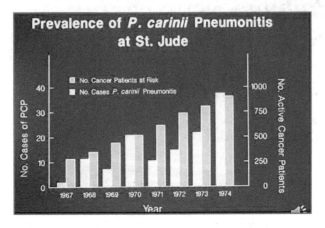

FIG. 14-B: Incidence and prevalence of PCP at St. Jude 1967-1974.

FIG. 14-B shows the incidence and prevalence of PCP during the early years at St. Jude. The yellow bars show the number of cases of PCP and the blue bars show the number of cancer patients at risk per year at St. Jude. You can see the epidemic had only begun when the CDC investigation occurred in 1967, 1968 and 1969. During my first year in 1970 there were 20 cases and by 1974 some 40 cases occurred annually. This increase was related to the number of cancer patients at risk.

Because of the large number of histologically diagnosed patients at one institution and the superb pathologists Warren Johnson, M.D. and Robert Price, M.D. and Cardio-Pulmonologist S. K. (Sam) Sanyal, MBBS we were able to clearly delineate the clinical features of PCP in more than 100 immunocompromised children with cancer. The clinical pattern was that of a sudden onset of fever, tachypnea and hypoxia. The chest radiograph showed diffuse bilateral alveolar disease, beginning in the lower lobes and progressing to upper lobes, with eventual lung whiteout, cyanosis and death. A specific diagnosis required demonstration of the organism in lung tissue obtained by biopsy or autopsy.

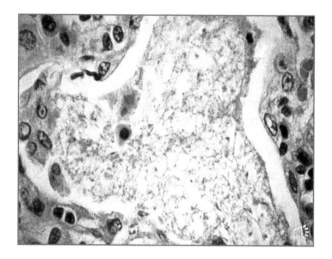

FIG. 14-C: Biopsy stained with hematoxylin and eosin.

FIG. 14-C shows a biopsy stained with standard hematoxylin and eosin stain. The alveolar space is filled with a foamy protein-aceous exudate with only a few reactive alveolar macrophages, but no organisms are seen.

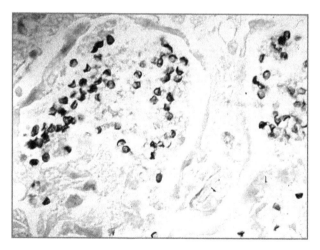

FIG. 14-D: Biopsy stained with Gomori-Grocott showing brown-black P. carinii cysts.

When the same specimen is stained with Gomori-Grocott methenamine silver nitrate the alveolar space is found filled with brown-black cysts of *P. carinii*. I think you can appreciate that if a needle were inserted into this tissue and a drop of fluid aspirated, one would likely find the organism. So we utilized a transthoracic pulmonary needle aspirate technique for the diagnosis of PCP, thus avoiding open-lung or transbronchial biopsies. The procedure proved to be highly useful for this purpose **(FIG. 14-E).**

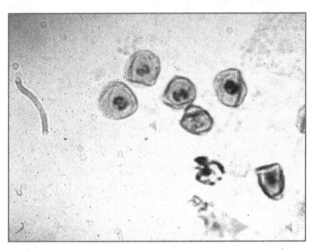

FIG. 14-E: Shows an aspirate stained with Grocott-Gomori method.

Unfortunately, we were able to delineate the natural course of PCP in children with cancer. We had 15 children with PCP for whom treatment could not be obtained in time **(FIG. 14-F)**. By the end of two weeks 50% of patients had died and by the end of six weeks all had died. We reported that without treatment PCP was a universal fatal infection in immunosuppressed children, once pneumonitis had become visible by chest radiograph.

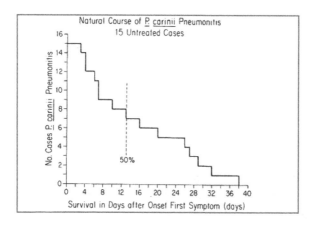

FIG. 14-F: Survival rates without treatment.

By 1974 St. Jude was entering a somewhat stressful mode. We were seeing 20 to 40 cases of PCP per year. They required intensive care and prolonged management. It was the most frequent cause of death for patients in remission, while other fatal opportunistic infections occurred predominantly in patients in relapse with neutropenia. It affected some of the oncology research protocols to the point adequate analysis of data was not possible. The parents were afraid. They were well aware of the circumstances and often referred to PCP as the "St. Jude Plague." We began to see a decrease in patient referrals, with some physicians apologizing for referring their patients elsewhere because of PCP. I recall at a staff meeting Dr. Pinkel raised the possibility of stopping all admissions to the hospital until the problem could be resolved.

Now, that's the background and this is where the lecture begins.

Research Leading to Resolution of PCP at St. Jude

What I hope to do now is to recognize the importance of an experimental animal model in the discovery and development of methods for the prevention and treatment of PCP in humans. Over the years we used this rat model for many other studies but here I shall only deal with our studies for prevention and treatment of the disease. I have provided an attachment with references to most of the other studies as well as to publications of the data mentioned here. **SEE APPENDIX 1.**

We continually searched the world literature for even the smallest morsel of information about *P. carinii*. Publications were sparse in the early 1970s. Fortunately, I ran across an obscure article published in 1955 by Weller in Germany. For some reason it had been published in a somewhat inappropriate journal, *Z. Kinderchir* .(The European Journal of Pediatric Surgery). Weller had attempted to infect rats with *P. carinii* by inoculating them intranasally with a suspension of infected lung. After a period of observation nothing happened and none became infected. He next pretreated rats with cortisone acetate, a newly discovered Compound F that suppressed immune responses, and then inoculated them intranasally with the suspension of *P. carinii*-infected lung. Subsequently all of the animals became infected with PCP.

Fortunately, Weller went one step further and added another group of animals to his study, a teaching moment for the use of controls. In this third group he administered the cortisone immunosuppression but did **not** inoculate them with *P. carinii.* Surprisingly, they became heavily infected with PCP, similar to the second group that had been inoculated with the organism. Weller eventually concluded that the rat population was probably latently infected with *P. carinii* in nature and if the host defenses became compromised the organism might replicate to create a disease state. Indeed, that was the case as other investigators have confirmed.

It occurred to us Weller's rat experiments might provide a resource for us to utilize in development of a method to prevent and treat PCP in humans. A first question to be resolved was, "Is the cortisone immunosuppressed rat representative of human disease?" A later study by Frankel, *et al* also showed cortisone immunosuppression would provoke PCP. However, no studies had compared the animal infection directly to the spectrum of disease in man. Precise similarities must be demonstrated to consider the immunosuppressed rat with PCP as highly representative model of human disease.

We obtained some Sprague-Dawley rats from Charles River, randomized littermates into two groups, gave one group cortisone acetate for six weeks and the other group received no drug. At the end of the study autopsies of the lungs showed PCP in all the cortisone-treated and no PCP in the control animals. The clear-cut all or none endpoint was impressive. In subsequent studies we continued to use the 6 to 7 week course of immunosuppression because we felt this prolonged course assured us of the easily discernible end point of 90 to 100 % with PCP

Because of the urgent need to prevent PCP in our patients at St. Jude we elected to seek an immunoprophylaxis approach with vaccine development. We harvested *P. carinii* cysts and trophozoites by bronchoalveolar lavage, prepared a whole cell vaccine in Freund's adjuvant, and immunized normal rats to achieve IgG antibody titers of 1:256. Upon challenge with cortisone immunosuppression the vaccinated rats succumbed to PCP at rates equal to the unvaccinated controls. These results came as no great surprise because by this time we had found that most patients had detectable antibody to *P. carinii* at the time of onset of PCP. Also, many cancer patients without PCP had detectable antibody to *P. carinii*.

Furthermore, we had recently studied a series of normal healthy infants and children being followed in Dr. Paul Zee's Nutrition Clinic at St. Jude and found progressive acquisition of antibody occurred after birth and by age four years 75% had detectable antibody to *P. carinii*. These findings suggested that immunoprophylaxis would not be effective, so we abandoned the vaccine studies and turned to developing a chemoprophylaxis approach and the search for an antimicrobial drug for PCP.

We reasoned that if we administered a test drug during the period of cortisone immunosuppression and at the end of 6 to 7 weeks no organisms could be found in the lungs, we could conclude that the drug was active against PCP. We then began to screen a number of drugs, focusing on antimalarial compounds and folate antagonists. At this time there was general agreement with Carini, Chagas, the Delano's' and others that *P. carinii* was a protozoan, similar to *Trypanosoma* and *Plasmodium* species.

To make a long story short we found that the drug combination Trimethoprim-Sulfamethoxazole (TMP-SMZ) was highly effective in the animal experiments. The drug was in clinical development in Europe as an antibiotic for the treatment of bacterial infections of the urinary tract. We included it in our screen because Dr. Alex Steigman, a colleague from my days in Louisville, had mentioned to me that there was some evidence to suggest that the combination might also have some anti-malarial activity. Trimethoprim inhibits dihydrofolate reductase the enzyme that reduces dihydrofolic acid to tetrahydrofolic acid an early stage in the process leading to the formation of purines and eventually DNA of certain bacteria and parasites. Sulfamethoxazole acts competitively to inhibit the incorporation of para-aminobenzoic acid (PABA) into dihydrofolate. So, with the drug combination we found that 15 of the 15 control animals that received cortisone and no TMP-SMZ died with PCP; whereas, none of the 15 rats given cortisone plus TMP-SMZ prophylactically had any evidence of *P. carinii in the* lungs at autopsy. When 15 rats were allowed to develop PCP and TMP-SMZ then begun therapeutically, 9 recovered, compared to none of an untreated group. Pentamidine was also evaluated for prophylaxis but found ineffective because of severe toxicity to the animals.

The results of the animal studies led us to move rapidly to clinical trials. By designing clinical trials similar to the animal studies we availed ourselves of opportunities to validate the cortisone-treated rat as an animal model for human disease. The fact that the drug combination had undergone phase I to III studies in Europe as an antibiotic for bacterial urinary tract infections allowed us to move quickly into clinical trials in the United States for its uses as an anti-PCP drug. Of course, at the time TMP-SMZ had never reached FDA approval for any use in the United States. However, clinical trials were underway in the U. S. A. to evaluate TMP-SMZ for the treatment of bacterial infections of the urinary and upper respiratory tracts.

The ownership of TMP-SMZ was shared between Burroughs

Wellcome where George Hitchings and Trudy Ellion had synthesized trimethoprim, the pyrimidine component, and Hoffman La Roche, where sulfamethoxazole had been in use for many years as a long-acting and safe sulfonamide. They were combined because of pharmacologic similarities as well as possible synergistic effects for some infections.

At St. Jude we were able to obtain an IND through Hoffman La Roche to evaluate TMP-SMZ in comparison to pentamidine isethionate for the treatment of children with cancer and documented PCP. We randomized 50 children with cancer and PCP to receive either TMP-SMZ orally or pentamidine isethionate, intramuscularly for the treatment of documented PCP.

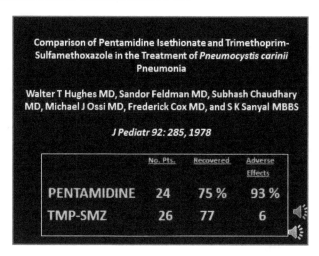

FIG. 14-G: Comparison of TMP-SMZ and Pentamidine at St. Jude.

At the end of the study three-fourths of each group had recovered from the specific treatment. The difference was in the analysis of adverse drug effects which occurred in 6% of the TMP-SMZ and 93% of the pentamidine group.

Soon after the onset of the study we had reason to believe that TMP-SMX was effective against PCP, because some cases were recovering with TMP-SMZ alone; our natural course studies had shown that no one recovers from PCP without effective treatment.

This gave us sufficient encouragement to develop a protocol to begin a large prophylaxis study evaluating TMP-SMZ vs. placebo in a double-blind study at St. Jude and I'll give you the results of this study shortly. But first let me comment on the format of some of the figures to follow.

I want to acknowledge the many people at St. Jude who took part in these studies over a period of several decades. In order to do so I have formatted the figures based on publications of the data. The title of the article is at the top, followed by the authors/investigators, name and date of the journal and the box at the bottom contains the bottom-line results. So, please give attention and recognition to the authors. These references are also listed in **APPENDIX 1.**

I will comment also that all the co-authors in the first study were first generation Infectious Diseases Fellows, except for **Sam Sanyal**. They included **Drs. Sandor Feldman, Subash Chaudhaury, Mike Ossi and Fred Cox,** all of whom have now retired from distinguished careers in the field of Pediatric Infectious Diseases. I am very proud of them all. **Sam Sanyal** had already completed a fellowship at Yale University in Pediatric Cardiology before coming to St. Jude. We recruited him to develop a cardiology-pulmonology intensive care unit at St. Jude for supportive care of critically ill patients and to investigate physiological aspects of PCP. This ICU was unique among cancer hospitals in the early 1970s, when heroic measures were not commonplace in terminal cancer care. Sam established a state-of-the art ICU at St. Jude that now comprises a central core of service. **Dr. Sanyal** pursued several scholarly studies on the cardio-pulmonary aspects of PCP (see references).

The randomized, double blind, placebo-controlled chemo-prophylaxis study enrolled 160 patients at high risk for PCP **(FIG. 14-H).** Of the 80 patients randomized to receive a placebo during the two-year study, 17 (20%) were found to have had PCP, while none of the 80 patients given TMP-SMZ orally each day acquired the infection. It was a happy day at St. Jude when the code was broken and these results revealed. We were already prepared to begin institution-wide TMP-SMZ prophylaxis for all St. Jude patients at risk because during the second year of the study the incidence of PCP dropped presumably because of the TMP-SMZ arm of the study.

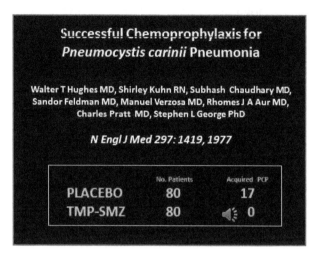

FIG. 14-H: Chemoprophylaxis study with TMP-SMZ.

Quick meetings, planning and discussions took place on predominantly face-to-face basis with Hematology-Oncology colleagues to administer TMP-SMZ to all St. Jude patients at risk for PCP. All were in favor without a single exception. We had excellent data tabulated (hand-written tables) from the past, on the incidence of PCP in each cancer category at St. Jude that would serve as a guide. TMP-SMZ had been approved by the FDA for the treatment of bacterial infections of the urinary tract under the trade names of **Bactrim**[R] for Hoffman La Roche and **Septra**[R] for Burroughs-Wellcome. So, what could go wrong? The call came from the Chief Pharmacist, "Hey Walter, bit of a problem here. We're getting prescriptions from the doctors for TMP-SMZ in a dosage for PCP prophylaxis. This is not an FDA-approved dose nor is this an FDA-approved indication. You know that we can't fill them. What to do?"

"How long will it take us to get FDA approval?" I asked while knowing the answer.

"Oh, two to five years if all goes well."

"I'll get back to you, I replied." Bedrock for St. Jude since its beginning was the Clinical Trials Committee, the forerunner of the Internal Review Board, established by Dr. Donald Pinkel, with the opening of the hospital to assure that no study, no experimental drug, no procedure and even no survey would involve a St. Jude patient without approved protocols and informed consent of patients and parents. Nothing short of this would be acceptable, even though my ID colleague suggested sending our patients to physicians in private practice who could easily write prescriptions for Bactrim and Septra for prophylaxis. So, we devised a plan that would allow us to proceed almost as planned.

Within a week we wrote and had approved by a special meeting of the Clinical Trials Committee a protocol for a study entitled "Evaluation of Unstructured Delivery of TMP-SMZ Prophylaxis in patients at high risk for PCP." A St. Jude investigator could enroll any patient for PCP prophylaxis without structured guidelines. An end point in this observational study was the number of cases per year of PCP occurring within the patient population at St. Jude. The aim was to evaluate how well physicians would use TMPSMZ prophylaxis for children with cancer. PCP prophylaxis was then applied to high-risk patients from 1977 until present time (38 yrs. later).

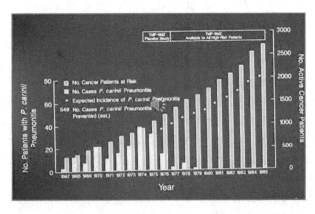

FIG. 14-I: Prevalence and incidence of Pneumocystis carinii pneumonia at St. Jude from 1967 to 1985.

FIG. 14-I shows a panoramic view of the incidence of PCP at St. Jude over a twenty-year period. As can be seen the TMP-SMZ prophylaxis quickly eradicated PCP from St. Jude and not a single case occurred over the ensuing five years. The white dots on the graph show the number of PCP cases that would have been expected to occur without prophylaxis, based on incidence from prior years. For example, from 1977 to 1985, 549 cases of PCP were prevented at St. Jude alone. Other centers repeated our studies, found similar results and PCP prophylaxis began to be used elsewhere.

Although our problem with PCP was seemingly becoming resolved, something just didn't seem right. The results were just too good. I was not accustomed to such success. Why had we not had a single case in five years? TMP-SMZ was static and not 'cidal so we were not likely eradicating *P. carinii* from the environment. These children were often very sick and sometimes missed several days of medication. It finally occurred to us that we might be using more TMP-SMZ, or using it more frequently, than needed.

Going back to the animal model Bessie Smith and I gave one group of rats TMP-SMZ daily and the other group TMP-SMZ only three days a week (Mon., Tues., and Wed.) and a third group received no TMP-SMZ during six weeks of cortisone immunosuppression. Both daily and three days a week TMP-SMZ was totally effective in PCP prevention, while all of untreated controls became infected. Thus, less than one-half our dose of TMP-SMZ was totally effective in PCP prophylaxis.

Because to date the animal model had been highly predictive of human disease, we elected to undertake another clinical trial. With the collaboration of hematology-oncology colleagues, we randomized children with cancer at high risk for PCP to receive TMP-SMZ either daily or only three consecutive days per week over a two-year period. The results **(FIG.14-J)** showed that TMP-SMZ three days a week was just as effective as daily administration of the drug. However, oral candidiasis and systemic fungal infections were significantly less frequent in the three-day a week group.

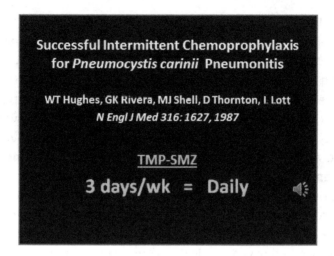

FIG. 14-J: Comparison of daily vs. three-days-a-week TMP-SMZ prophylaxis.

Studies by other investigators have subsequently shown similar results and the three-days-a-week regimen has been accepted into general use.

At this point it seemed that reasonably satisfactory methods were available for the treatment and prevention of PCP in the immunocompromised patient and I began a new phase of my career. My interest in *Pneumocystis carinii* was problem solving much more than scientific curiosity. I felt I had accomplished what I had set out to do and left this fertile field for basic research to the curious scientists. As I had moved away from Tularemia in the past, maybe I should now focus on my original interest of fungi. Little did I know that I had only experienced half my story of **Pneumocystis** pneumonia. Chapter 17 chronicles **the rest of the story!**

Chronologically, I must interrupt my story of *Pneumocystis* pneumonia at this point in 1977 to tell you about another major change in my life, as well as for Jeanette, Carla, Greg and Chris.

The year 1977 was one of change. The young faculty of 27 people when I joined in 1969 was growing up fast, now 96 people, gaining more and more notoriety and were now beginning to be picked upon. The number of active patients had increased from 1,065 in 1969 to 3,370 in 1977, and the annual budget went from $3,182,762 to $15,218,830, respectively. Don Pinkel had been pulled away to be Chairman of the Dept. Pediatrics and Physician-in-Chief of the Children's Hospital at the Medical College of Wisconsin and Joe Simone had accepted a position at Stanford University to head the Pediatric Hematology/Oncology Division. Others were in the process of change, not because of dissatisfaction with St. Jude but because of their meritorious work.

I also had offers and had begun to give thought to the future. We had successfully resolved the problem of *Pneumocystis carinii* pneumonia; the new six-story building was complete and in operation and we had accrued an excellent group of faculty and trainees in the Infectious Diseases Service listed below. By 1977 I was 47 years old and had yet to gain a desire for an academic Chairmanship or Dean, and had no interest in moving to a higher leadership level at St. Jude. However, I was always pleased to be considered for a position elsewhere - I have an ego like all other humans. Nevertheless, I regularly and kindly declined offers that came to me without ever going for a visit, because I was happy at St. Jude.

For some reason, possibly ego, when I received a call from Dr. John Littlefield, Chairman of the Department of Pediatrics at The Johns Hopkins University School of Medicine, inviting me to be a candidate for the director of the Division of Infectious Diseases in his Department, at Johns Hopkins Hospital I became interested. I recalled the enjoyable first two years of married life Jeanette and I spent in Maryland, near Baltimore; my friend from Louisville, Dr. Alex Haller now a famous Pediatric Surgeon at Hopkins; and my acquaintance with a young junior faculty member, Dr. Richard Moxon, in the Division I was being asked to head. A year or so earlier Richard had come to St. Jude to spend a week on our service to learn about opportunistic infections. He had recently come out of a Fellowship at Harvard and Boston Children's Hospital and I was very impressed with his potential.

The interview at Hopkins was a visit to the history of Medicine in America, walking the halls tread by Osler, Halstead, Welsh,

Blalock, Taussig and many others. The massive medical complex of the medical school, hospital and the famous Harriet Lane Children's Center were impressive. Dr. Littlefield was a gracious, intellectual and compassionate Chairman who toured me through a two-day visit of the Children's Medical Center (CMSC) and dynamic faculty. After the visit he offered me the endowed Eudowood Professorship of Pediatric Infectious Diseases and Director of the Division of Infectious Diseases, an increase in salary, liberal space for research laboratories and additional faculty in the Division. Back home Jeanette expressed no strong opinion with her usual "Whatever you think is best, will be fine with me." Carla was graduating from high school and would be away in college. My main concern was Greg who would be moving for his senior high school year, the worst time to move, but Greg voiced no opposition to the change. Chris had changed schools earlier in Memphis and did well with a change.

So, in 1977 we moved to Baltimore. In retrospect, I believe I realized some ego gratification progressing from a Tennessee farm boy at the Home Place in Bradley County to a prestigious Professorship at The Johns Hopkins University School of Medicine. My world was now undergoing further expansion, but back to the traditional academic scene.

CHAPTER 15

The Johns Hopkins University School of Medicine – 1977 to 1981

On my first day at Hopkins I parked on Broadway Ave. at about 7 AM, walked up the brick drive to the main entrance **(FIG.15-A)** and moved with the arriving young doctors, nurses, students and visitors through the opened massive oak doors into the hall of the "Dome".

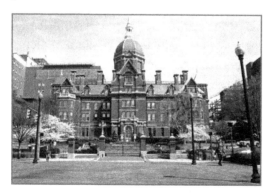

FIG. 15-A: Entrance to The Johns Hopkins University Medical Center through the original hospital building (circa 1898). Tops of the 14-acre building complex of hospital and medical school are seen from behind the iconic entry (Courtesy Johns Hopkins Hospital).

Just inside the Dome was the massive 11-foot marble *Christus* statue by Bertel Thorvaldsen **(FIG. 15-B)** with the beckoning inscription, *"Come unto me all ye who are weary and heavy laden and I will give you rest."* I paused a moment to reflect back only seven years ago when I passed another marble statue of similar dimensions and prominence but of **St. Jude Thaddeus (FIG. 13-A)** at the entrance to my new job at St. Jude Children's Research Hospital. Aside from the Cerra marble of their statues I could think of few simiarities of the two institutions.

Wow! What a change I thought. I could not imagine two more strikingly different worlds I had entered. The first, a two-story concrete block and stucco structure over Bayou Gayoso in Memphis with its 30 beds and full-time faculty of 27 unknown venturesome pioneers, less than 45 years of age "wingin' it" into dreams of Camelot. And now the second, a massive world-renowned 1,000 bed Johns Hopkins Hospital with a professional staff of some 400 full-time faculty, 600 part time members and 400 interns and residents along with the large 14-acre medical complex of the Johns Hopkins University School of Medicine. This is where in 1910 Abraham Flexner (chapter 12), a recent Hopkins undergraduate and humble school teacher from Louisville, KY, pointed to this institution as a model for the future of medical education, and it was so. From under this dome came the legacy of American Medicine from Sir William Osler, William Halstead, William Welch, Howard Kelly, and others to a century of doctors, teachers, scientists, researchers , Nobel Laureates, and others. Nevertheless, in my own mind I considered the two institutions in equal esteem, thinking of the accomplishments of St. Jude in its first decade compaired to the first decade at Hopkins. I thought St. Jude will catch up.

Feeling a bit **heavy ladened** I touched the foot of **CHRISTUS** in passing as millions had done before me requesting Divine help and moved through the exits behind the statue into the freeway of hospital traffic on my way to the nearby elevators to the Children's Medical-Surgical Center (CMSC) where the offices and laboratories of my Division of Infectious Diseases were located on the 11th floor.

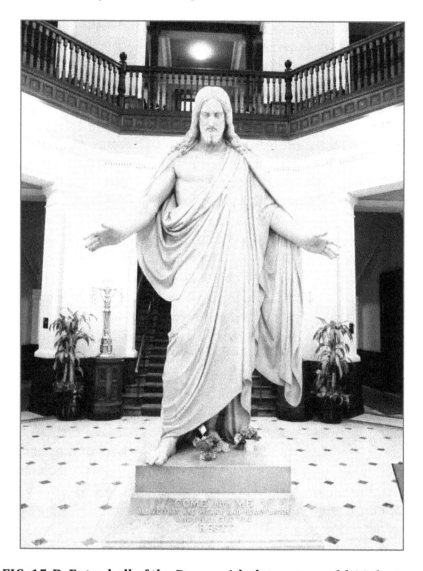

FIG. 15-B: Entry hall of the Dome with the century old 11-foot marble CHRISTUS statue by Bertel Thorvaldsen (Courtesy Art Anderson, panoramino.com).

At 7:30 AM I stepped off the elevator on CMSC-11. All was quiet and I was the only person around. I was familiar with the domain from previous visits and easily found my office, which was open.

I closed the door and sat in my big chair still thinking of my new job. On my desk were new crisp copies of the *Hospital Telephone Directory* and *The Johns Hopkins University Circular* (catalogue). Thumbing through these pages I read the names of my new colleagues and occupants of 11-story CMSC. Here is the Department of Pediatrics, comprised of more than 250 full-time faculty, 13 of whom hold full professorships. Of the 13 Professors, five hold named, endowed positions and I am privileged to be one of them as the Eudowood Professor of Pediatric Infectious Diseases and Director of the Division of Pediatric Infectious Diseases.

I mention this here for my children and grandchildren who are asking, "How did he do that?" How did the little farm boy on the Home Place in Bradley County, TN come to sit in this office at 47 years of age? All I can say is that I don't know, and that I did not ask for it. Never did I apply for this position and never did I ever voice an interest in recruitment for the job. That was just never a Hughes thing to do. Somewhere in chapters 1 through 15 may be the answer. Perhaps the most difficult decision of my life was deciding to come here to Hopkins for my future, rather than staying at St. Jude.

This morning, I thought of my good friend Joe Simone who left St. Jude the day I did to take a similar position as Professor and Division Director at the Stanford University School of Medicine in California. I expect Joe's somewhat humble beginnings led him to musings like mine. By whatever means we got to where we were now, I must conclude St. Jude (i.e., the people of) had a lot to do with it.

On my starting day at St. Jude I also had a desk and chair (small) but that was all. Today, seven years later, I inherit the efforts of the former Director, **Dr. David Carver,** who had accepted the position of Pediatrician-in Chief of the famous Hospital for Sick Children (circa 1875) in Toronto. My office was large with adjoining two- desk secretarial office and experienced young secretarial assistants. Extending down the hall were three offices, one of which was occupied by the young **Dr. Richard Moxon,** Assistant Professor of Pediatrics, who had visited me at St. Jude. I would recruit occupants for the other offices. Laboratories and animal facilities were also conveniently located on CMSC-11. Adjacent to our Division was that of Pediatric Immunology, headed by **Jerry Winkelstein, MD,** an ideal colleague for our group. The hall in front of my office led into Blalock Building and the location for the Department of Medicine, Division of Infectious Diseases, for which a Director was being sought.

Now, you and others should be asking, what is Hughes going to do here at Hopkins? I had clearly in mind what I wished to accomplish with the Division of Infectious Diseases. My **Five-Year Strategic Plan** included the establishment of a **Comprehensive Postdoctoral Fellowship Training Program in Pediatric Infectious Diseases**, encompassing input from the university-wide resources and to foster the establishment of Infectious Diseases as a subspecialty of Pediatrics. " Big deal! How dull", you think after the **Pneumocystis** eradication stuff at St. Jude. So, I need to explain circumstances of the day.

In 1977 Infectious Diseases had not been established as a subspecialty of Pediatrics. The American Academy of Pediatrics recognized for accreditation only subspecialties in Cardiology, Allergy and Immunology, Endocrinology and Neonatology. Of course there was no formal training program for pediatricians who wished to specialize in Infectious Diseases. Rather, one must serve an apprentice-"Fellowship" with a specific individual or academic institution. Many of these were outstanding experiences and led to leaders in the field. However, the experiences were narrow and unique with no comprehensive program aimed to train a board-certified subspecialist as Pediatric Infectious Diseases. I had designed a comprehensive two-year fellowship program to cover experience in the basic research laboratory, clinical aspects of special problems of infections in children, pharmacodynamics, epidemiology, microbiology, hospital epidemiology and nosocomial infections, biostatistics and experimental design, etc. which I hoped to implement at Hopkins. Hopefully, this would serve as a forerunner of a new accredited subspecialist in Pediatric Infectious Diseases.

At the time I went to Hopkins the most authoritative group in Pediatric Infectious Diseases was the **Committee on Infectious Diseases of the American Academy of Pediatrics.** This committee since 1938 had published its **Report,** providing expert recommendations in the area of infectious diseases and immunization, often referred to as **The Redbook,** or the Pediatricians "Bible." In **1977** the 18th edition was published with **Alex J. Steigman, M.D**. (my first boss in Louisville) as Editor. Membership of the Committee included the great **Martha Yow, MD, Chair, Samuel Katz, MD, a former Chair, Ernesto Jaimes, MD, David Carver, MD, Henry Cramblett, M.D., Thomas Frothingham, MD, Vincent Fulginniti, MD, Samuel Gotoff, MD, Walter Hughes, MD, Jerome Klein, MD, Paul Quie, MD, Richard Stiehm, MD, Saul Krugman and Edward Mortimer, MD**. The attitude of the American Academy of Pediatrics at this time was that infectious diseases was so much a part of general pediatrics, a subspecialty was not warranted. However, several of us were concerned about the emerging problems with infectious diseases that would likely require dedicated expertise and research.

My immediate task was to fill the empty offices. Fortunately, I had been blessed with **Dr. Richard Moxon** already on board and ready to develop his own career as well as that of our Division. He came from a fellowship at Harvard University and Boston Children's' Hospital where he worked on an *Haemophilus influenzae* vaccine. Richard wished to continue work on *H. influenzae*. Here some serendipity arose at Hopkins because two faculty members in the Department of Microbiology, **Dan Nathans, MD** and **Hamilton Smith, MD** were investigating the endonucleases (restriction enzymes) of *H. influenzae* to split DNA sequences. Richard arranged a collaboration and I approved allocation of time for this affiliation and he obtained NIH grant support. This was the type of interdepartmental and interdisciplinary interaction I had hoped to foster at Hopkins as I did at St. Jude. Of course, Nathans and Smith were awarded the Nobel Prize in 1978 and Richard's role in our Division was meritorious. To move a bit ahead at this time, lest I forget,

Richard eventually became Professor and Director of the Hopkins Division after I left. Soon thereafter he was appointed as Professor and Chairman, Department of Pediatrics at Oxford University and John Radcliff Hospital in UK. At his invitation I later spent a week as Visiting Professor with him at Oxford University and he in turn came back to St. Jude as a special speaker (as recent as 2014}. Richard has been a dear friend for more than 38 years.

My first fresh recruit was **Robert H. Yolken, MD**. I had interviewed a few candidates but none was precisely what I sought. I wanted someone like Richard. On the first visit I knew Bob Yolken was my choice (Richard agreed). Bob was a graduate of Harvard Medical School and had completed a residency in Pediatrics at Yale University Medical Center and had been in a research program of enteric viral infections at the National Institute of Allergy and Infectious Diseases in Bethesda. When Bob moved in on CMSC-11 as Assistant Professor, his space was immediately filled with specimens, equipment and people and he was off to a running start, which never slowed. During my time at Hopkins Bob was an excellent faculty member with loyalty to our objectives and many research contributions and grant support. He later became Professor and Director of the Division of Pediatric Infectious Diseases and is currently the Theodore and Vada Stanley Distinguished Professor of Neurovirology in Pediatrics at Johns Hopkins and chairs the Division of Pediatric Neurovirology .

In 1977 the Hospital-acquired Infection Control Program at the 1000-bed Johns Hopkins Hospital was under auspices of Nursing and an Infection Control Committee. For more than two decades Infectious diseases acquired in hospitals were becoming a major problem worldwide to the extent that physician subspecialists were beginning to emerge as Hospital Epidemiologist. With the support of **Dr. Pat Charache**, Director of Clinical Microbiology Laboratories and serving as Director of Infectious Diseases in the Department of Medicine, we proposed to the Hospital Administrator, that Hopkins hire a physician Hospital Epidemiologist. I prepared data to show that not only would the position pay for itself but thousands of dollars would be saved in other ways. Wisely, the Administration approved the position and Pat and I were to search for candidates. If the recruit were an Internist he or she would be in the Division of Infectious Diseases in Medicine; if a Pediatrician, he or she would hold a faculty appointment in our Pediatric Division. Happily, the salary would come from the Hospital administration.

Somehow, I was blessed again by finding an ideal candidate, **Timothy R. Townsend, M.D.**, one of the first *bonefide* Pediatric Hospital Epidemiologists, easily appointed to the position and Assistant Professor of Pediatrics in our Division. As I write about Tim I realize I had recruited my new Division from the Boston bastion without even realizing it. Moxon, Yolken and Townsend were examples in my view of "Southern Gentlemen" from up north. Our interaction was enjoyable. I recall a Division faculty meeting on Tim's sailboat in Chesapeake Bay, where we could speak freely to each other and discuss institutional politics. Tim was a graduate of the University of Virginia School of Medicine, a resident in Pediatrics at St. Louis Children's' Hospital, a Fellow in Infectious Diseases at Channing Laboratory, Harvard Medical School and most recently a Fellow in Hospital Epidemiology at the University of Virginia. Of course, Tim became famous in his field and his contributions require a book on nosocomial infection and education. I suppose my selection of Tim was correct because he is still (2015), like Bob Yolken, on the faculty at Johns Hopkins in Baltimore.

The Chairman of the Department of Medicine, **Victor McKusik, MD**, asked me to become a member of his search committee for a Director of Infectious Diseases, Dept. of Medicine. The committee had been deliberating for some time and I was pleased to take part because the appointment would be important to our program in Pediatrics. Fortunately, soon thereafter the committee recommended **John G. Bartlett, MD**, who accepted the position and became my neighbor in Blalock down the hall from CMSC – 11. I recall John in my office at 7 am soon after arrival asking where he might get a coffee maker with capacity of 25 cups per day. He usually arrived at 5 am.

To accomplish the "ideal" postdoctoral training program that I had in mind required two elements: organization of resources and funding. A training grant from the National Institute of Allergy and Infectious Diseases would suffice for both needs. My application proposed to train specialists in the field of Pediatric Infectious Diseases for positions in academic medicine and research. Based in our Division the curriculum encompassed rotations through clinical consultation services at CMSC, the Clinical Microbiology Diagnostic Laboratories under Dr. Pat Charache and Dr. William Merz; Biostatistics, Epidemiology and Experimental Design courses in the School of Public Health and Hygiene under Dr. Leon Gordis; Immunology with Dr. Jerry Winkelstein, our next door neighbor on CMSC; Hospital Epidemiology with Townsend, options for electives; and the second year would be dedicated to a laboratory-based research project under the mentorship of a faculty member. Fortunately, the grant was approved and fully funded for the next four years. From the beginning our trainees in Pediatric Infectious Diseases were excellent and have made a significant impact in the field. The program continues some four decades later with basically the same structure.

FELLOWS:

The earliest **Fellows** beginning with my tenure at Hopkins have now made their marks and I can recall them fondly. I believe the first was **Stuart P. Adler**, MD who had come through Hopkins as an undergraduate, medical student and Pediatric resident and had recently spent a special research project with Dr. Dan Nathans and Hamilton Smith in the Department of Microbiology working with *H. influenzae* endonucleases. A year into the fellowship Nathans and Smith received the Nobel Award in Medicine and acknowledged in an institutional convocation the input of Stuart in their work. After the fellowship in 1979 he joined the faculty at the Medical College of Virginia in Richmond and later became Director of the Division of Pediatric Infectious Diseases where he spent his career as a leader in the field of cytomegalovirus.

Robert Leggiadro, MD came from a Pediatric residency at Nassau County Hospital in Long Island, New York. When I first met with him in Baltimore, he asked, "Where are the palm trees?" (jokingly) because this was the farthest South he had ever been. After the Fellowship Bob spent a productive academic career as Director of Pediatric infectious Diseases and later as a Chairman of Departments of Pediatrics in New York and New Jersey. Importantly, he later searched for palm trees in Memphis as Professor of Pediatrics at the University of Tennessee College of Medicine and Consultant to my Department at St. Jude Children's Research Hospital. While Memphis has yet to grow Palm trees, Bob and Patti became close life-long friends of Jeanette and myself.

Other early Fellows recruited during my four-tenure at Hopkins were **Leonard R. Krilov, MD, Lorry G. Rubin, MD,** and **C. James Corrall, MD.** Both Lenni Krilov and Lorry Rubin returned to New York for prestigious careers in Pediatric Infectious Diseases. Leonard is Chief of Pediatric Infectious Diseases at North Shore University Hospital and Lorry is Chief of Pediatric Infectious Diseases, Schneider Children's Hospital and Professor of Pediatrics at Albert Einstein College of Medicine in New York. They have both made significant contributions to the field of Infectious Diseases. Jim Corrall went to University of Southern Illinois in Peoria as Associate Professor of Pediatrics.

RESIDENTS:

If you asked anyone at the Johns Hopkins Hospital in 1977 what is the most important position in the institution, whether in Pediatrics, Medicine, Surgery, or other, the resounding reply would be, "The Chief Resident". This stems from the fact that since Osler, the house staff of residents and interns was in charge of the patients. Their management was the ultimate responsibility of the residents and the Chief Resident was their commander. The Faculty held a more advisory role and would make daily rounds with their team of residents, Pediatric residents in my case, listen to their case presentations at the bedside and be expected to make some wise comments.

One of the first people I met after arriving in Baltimore was **Dr. Dennis Stokes**, Chief Resident in Pediatrics. We met not on the ward but on the bus. A shuttle bus circulated from the Homewood Campus of Johns Hopkins University near the residential suburbs and the downtown medical campus. From my house I could walk a short distance and ride the bus with other faculty and students to my office. Dennis introduced himself to me and we sat together for a brief chat. He had completed his Pediatric Residency at Hopkins a couple of years earlier, gone to Boston for a Fellowship in Pulmonology at Harvard and had just returned to spend the next year as Chief Resident in Pediatrics. He originally came from Kentucky and I soon concluded he was my kind of person. He became interested in *Pneumocystis carinii* pneumonia and we collaborated on studies at Hopkins and a few years later when I returned to St. Jude we were able to recruit Dennis to head the Intensive Care Unit and Pulmonology program. After moves to head programs at Vanderbilt and Dartmouth Universities he eventually returned to Memphis to head Pulmonary at Le Bonheur Children's Hospital, the University of Tennessee College of Medicine and St. Jude. Now in retirement he remains my close friend.

Two other Hopkins residents, for whom I had served as Faculty Attending staff ended up at St. Jude. **Dr. Victor Santana** and **Dr. Joe Mirro** became Pediatric Hematology/Oncologists and have had distinguished careers at St. Jude.

I must mention another Hopkins resident to whom I became attached. For several years the editors at W. B. Saunders Co., publisher of my book, **Pediatric Procedures,** had asked me to write a second edition and I refused because I had been too long away from the subject matter. However, their repeat request caused me to think of competent Hopkins resident as a co-author. I chose **Dr. E. Stephen Buescher**, gave him a copy of the book to look over and get back to me as to interest in the task. The next day he was in my office excited and anxious to get started. He wanted to replace all the illustrations with his own drawings; turns out art was his hobby. The year of the revision was delightful because of Steve's enthusiasm and sense of humor. He brought line drawings to life. I recall one of the editors called about one of them and said, "Dr. Hughes, the revised illustration of the human skeleton showing sites for bone marrow aspirates is satisfactory and we will allow the coon-skin cap and the high-top tennis shoes that Steve has added - we just ask that he removes the Adidas label from the shoes." As I had used my daughter Carla as a model for the first edition, Steve used his young son Geoff for the second edition **(FIG. 15-C, FIG. 15-D).** Steve completed a fellowship at the N.I.H. joined the faculty at the University of Texas Medical School in Houston as a Pediatric Infectious Diseases specialist and later was Professor of Pediatrics at Eastern Virginia Medical School in Norfolk, VA where he continues to be productive through research and teaching.

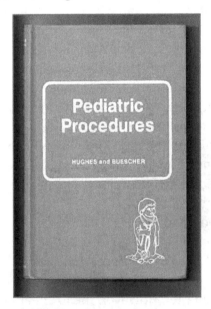

FIG. 15-C: Second Edition published in 1980 with Steve Buescher's artwork including son Geoffrey on cover.

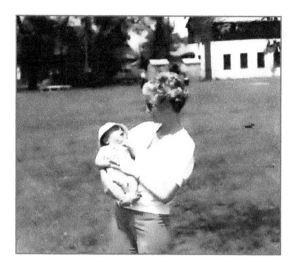

FIG. 15-D: Jeanette holding little Geoff Buescher at Johns Hopkins House-staff and Faculty July 4th Outing at Ft. McHenry on Chesapeake Bay.

Surely the most "ambidextrous" or "multidisciplinary" Pediatric Resident during my time at Hopkins was **David A. Kessler, MD.** Coming to Hopkins with a MD degree from Harvard and a JD degree from the University of Chicago, and while a resident at CMSC he worked as a consultant to Senator Orrin Hatch (R-Utah) on safety of food additives and the regulation of tobacco. His appointment as Commissioner of the Food and Drug Administration (FDA) in 1990 by President George H. W. Bush and again by President Bill Clinton was not surprising. His impact was phenomenal as the FDA leader. He kindly responded to my invitation to come to St. Jude in 1995 to deliver the John Erskine Lecture. He went on to become Dean of Yale School of Medicine in 1997 and later Dean and Vice-Chancellor at the University of California Medical School, San Francisco in 2003. Adequate recognition of Kessler would require another book.

I continue to recall the many residents, fellows and students with whom I had contact on CMSC during my four-year tenure there. All were outstanding and it saddens me not to be able to ramble on about them due to lack of pages and time (you know,

I'm 84 years old, nearing 85 years and can't dally too long at the keyboard). Nevertheless, I must mention one more. About the time I came to Hopkins in 1977, a new resident in Pediatric Neurosurgery arrived at CMSC, namely, **Benjamin S. Carson, MD,** at age 26 years. I recall him answering consultation requests for Pediatric patients on our service but more vividly I remember what I was told about this young African-American's devotion to Christian principles and his volunteer services to the nearby Black community. It was this that caused me to watch his career from the appointment at age 33 yrs. as the youngest Professor and Director, Division of Pediatric Neurosurgery at Johns Hopkins to present day when he is being supported nationally as a candidate for the President of the United States. I have often wondered about the relationship of **David Kessler** and **Ben Carson** as residents at CMSC. That would be a story!

PEDIATRIC INFECTIOUS DISEASES CLUB/ SOCIETY

A major event in the establishment of Pediatric Infectious Diseases as a subspecialty began in 1978, soon after I arrived at Hopkins due in part to the imagination and efforts of **Stanley Plotkin, MD.,** Director of Infectious Diseases, The Joseph Stokes. Jr. Research Institute, The Children's, Hospital of Philadelphia. Stanley recounts his original thoughts were to organize a "Club" of Pediatric Infectious Diseases specialists who knew each other through publications, but often had never met. He also, as did many others, considered Pediatric Infectious Diseases as a legitimate subspecialty. He thought if we could organize we might obtain recognition. Single-handed, Stanley organized the inaugural meeting of the "Pediatric Infectious Diseases Club" at the New York Hilton Hotel on April 27, 1978 of individuals across country who were his 'indivisible college' of PID specialists. I was included. The event was successful with 97 attendees paying of $7.50 per person for the four course dinner. From this historic event came many memorable annual meetings of the "Club" alongside national meetings allowing us to "bond'. The

"Club" grew and began to form plans for the future.

Formal bylaws of the Pediatric Infectious Diseases Club were developed and approved in 1983, requiring definition of membership, an Executive Committee and the election of a Secretary/Treasurer, a President and President-elect. **Dr. Stanley Plotkin** was designated as the **Founding Father** of the Pediatric Infectious Diseases Club (and later Society).

In 1983, **Karen Breese Hall, MD** was elected as the first **Secretary/Treasurer** and, **Walter Hughes, MD** was the first **President** of the Club/Society. The following are some abstracts from my Presidential Farewell talk at the end of 1984:

…"I was never sure why I was selected as the first President of the Infectious Diseases Club/Society, and even more unsure as to why I accepted the job. The challenge was a "Club" of about 200 members, with no bylaws, no budget or source of funds and the expectation of an annual national meeting with dinner. One-half the membership was in favor of drafting bylaws, changing the name from Club to Society, and establishing subspecialty Boards in Pediatric Infectious Diseases. The other half opposed these ventures. No one was undecided. Nevertheless, it was a fun group of bright, dedicated and opinionated Pediatricians with a pioneering spirit."

…"The members of the 1983-84 group were remarkable. They debated the issues, sent out surveys, repeated surveys, communicated with and without email and fax, drafted and re-drafted, begged for money, and enjoyed the climatic annual dinner meetings. Somehow, at the end of the two-year period we have changed the name from Club to Society, incorporated, established and approved the first set of bylaws, become tax-exempt, and initiated plans to pursue the establishment of Boards in Pediatric Infectious Diseases. Importantly, the Club spirit is greater than ever. The credit for these developments goes to the members, not the President."

It took another decade and the persistence and patience of **Dr. Sarah Long** and her Committee (**James Cherry, MD, Micheal A. Gerber, MD, Jerome O. Klein, MD, Georges Peter, MD**, and **Keith Powell, MD**) for their petition to the American Board of Pediatrics for subspecialty of Pediatric Infectious Diseases to be accepted and culminate in the first Board examination in 1994.

By 1997 the Pediatric Infectious Diseases Society had more than 900 members, was holding annual national meetings, publishing a monthly journal and the subspecialty of Pediatric Infectious Diseases was-well established. I was honored by the Society to be given the **Distinguished Physician Award** in company with others who contributed to this phase of Pediatric Infectious Diseases.

In subsequent years **a bit of serendipity** arose when St. Jude Children's Research Hospital became a designated venue for the Society's annual scientific forum where members and guests present research papers. This successful endeavor is now in its 14th year and must credited, not in any way to me, but to the efforts of **Elaine Tuomanen, MD,** who succeeded me as Chairman of the Department of Infectious Diseases at St. Jude, and is a world leader in the field of Infectious Diseases.

A PERSPECTIVE ON FAMILY AND CAREER

In this chapter I have rambled on about myself and my career at Hopkins. Now I must tell you about those most important to me, namely Jeanette, Carla, Greg and Chris. At the time of arrival in Baltimore we settled in a beautiful stone house built into the hillside on 5212 Springlake Way in Homeland overlooking some tiny lakes. Carla had graduated from Central High School and was enrolled as a freshman at the American University in nearby Washington, DC to major in Education and minor in Ballet. Greg had left Memphis at the time of his senior year in high school and was entering the senior year in a totally new class at the Lake Clifton High School, a large Baltimore high school. Chris was enrolled at Friends School, an old established private school in Baltimore City. Jeanette had suffered through the massive chores of moving household and family, finding a new home and placement of children in schools. Although she and I had enjoyed our two years in Maryland in 1957-59, circumstances in Baltimore in 1977 were different. The "southern" lifestyle we had come to appreciate in Memphis was lacking in Baltimore. I cannot recall the name of a neighbor and we were never able to find a Methodist Church to our liking. When Greg graduated and was accepted at the University of Maryland and the University of Memphis, he without hesitation chose the latter and moved to Memphis. Carla had also chosen to move back to Memphis and attend the University of Memphis. Chris excelled at Friends School academically and in sports but bore some intimidation of a southern boy up north. Jeanette persisted despite missing her close friends and family and lack of the friendly environment to which she had become accustomed. We moved to another neighborhood at 4312 St. Paul Street but with little improvement in lives.

After more than three years in Baltimore Jeanette and I came to the conclusion that we did not want to spend our lives in this city and that we might best make the move now rather than delay. Interestingly, my colleague Joe Simone had already returned to St. Jude to become the Deputy Director after a year at Stanford University in California. So, in 1981 I also returned to St. Jude as Member and Chairman of the Department of Infectious Diseases.

CHAPTER 16

House and Home

"I had rather be on my farm than be emperor of the world."
George Washington

"He is the happiest, be he king or peasant,
who finds peace in his home."
Johann Wolfgang von Goethe

During the fall and early winter of 1980 I was homeless in Baltimore. My departure date from Hopkins was to be January 1, 1981. In order to enroll Chris at the beginning of the school year Jeanette and he moved to Memphis in September and were staying in a guesthouse of our friends Dr. Cos and Sue Berard from St. Jude. When our Baltimore house sold I took a one-bedroom apartment across the street from Johns Hopkins Hospital. The Hopkins-owned facility was occupied predominantly by students, visitors to the university and others whom I was never able to identify.

At this point you are not to feel sorrow for poor Jeanette and Chris all alone in Memphis. You must have pity in your hearts for me, Walter, living alone in Hurd Hall. There is nothing good to say about it except for the occasions when my gracious colleagues at Hopkins brought me into their homes for dinners, etc. I recall Tim and Tonya Townsend serving Elvis Presley wine, just to cheer me up. Otherwise, days and nights were misery. I must say that at one point I concluded that every husband should be removed from his family for three months to live alone in order for him to truly appreciate the great blessings of his family.

For my children, grandchildren, great grandchildren and subsequent progeny I lament some of my woes while away from **a HUGHES FAMILY.** So, you husbands and husbands-to-be take notice!

My apartment neighbors remained unknown, without exception. Up and down the halls were robot-like, fast moving, forward gazing, backpacking, pale, younger people obviously intent on success. A 50 year old Professor in their presence was obviously out of place. So, I left early in the morning and returned late in the evening, spending time in my office where I was heavily pressed to complete grant reports and chapter manuscripts. I had meals in the dining room at Johns Hopkins Hospital.

The most miserable times were weekends. Jeanette had written clearly and specifically how to do my laundry. I first went to the laundry facilities in the basement of Hurd Hall on Saturday afternoon. Embarrassing!! As I entered three or four of the students waiting for washing machines stepped back and offered that I go ahead of them. This wasn't my way. Subsequently, what to do about my laundry became worrisome. Next week I took my bag of laundry far away to a Laundromat in Towson, where no one would know me. I had purchased the detergent that Jeanette had specified, had it in the bag with my dirty clothes so I would not forget it and entered the laundromat with the swagger of a seasoned user, like those adult men and women around me. What could go wrong? I even remembered to bring a pocket-full of quarters. The friendly Chinese lady attendant directed me to an available machine.

With gusto I dumped my stuff into the industrial washer, inserted two quarters, pushed start and took a seat to wait. By the time I sat and picked up a *Ladies Home Journal* magazine, a loud thumping noise came from my washer and the little Chinese lady came running to the rescue. The embarrassment was not that I had forgotten to take the box of detergent from my load but rather the humiliation that came in front of everyone when her shrill voice said, "Sir, you must take powder out of box." I never really mastered the laundry bit.

More painful than the daily chores of laundry, cleaning my room, shopping, paying bills, closing out utilities, were the lonely nights in my dark room without TV, video, texting, email. etc., thinking of Jeanette and Chris in Memphis. My little ten-dollar bedside radio was a close friend.

Jeanette's mission in Memphis included finding us a house to buy. For this task she was well prepared. This would be the 8th house we would purchase as our personal residence and it would not be the last.

For those who never knew us, some explanation is needed. From the first time we met Jeanette and I realized a common interest in houses and homes – there's a difference in the two, of course, but here I'll only deal with "house." I can't explain why we had a passion for houses, any more than why we passionately loved each other. It really doesn't matter why. I could reflect back to my childhood in my father's workshop in Bradley County, an interest in residential architecture (Chapters 3 and 7) and Jeanette's gardening with her mother and natural creative talent for colors and interior decoration, but as I have said it really doesn't matter why. It provided a strong bond for us and our family. Our "hobby" was the restoration of old homes and creative modifications of new houses. We **never** directed our interest to a recent practice of "flipping houses". Rather, we sought out an architecturally sound and appealing (to us) large old house in need of repair, purchased it for our residence, moved in and over time created the restoration, living there until some event or a new restoration challenge emerged. This was financially advantageous because we always sold for more than our investment and invested the profit in the next house. At one point Jeanette had gone to the University of Memphis for Real Estate courses, became a licensed Real Estate broker and joined a local firm but soon returned to our own home projects.

I am not just trying to appease Greg by acknowledging the wisdom of a philosophical Psychologist, but I think the following quotation by Bachelard defines remarkably well our focus on house as an important factor in the home and family.

"Of course, thanks to the house, a great many of our memories are housed, and if the house is a bit elaborate, if it has a cellar and a garret, nooks and corridors, our memories have refuges that are the more clearly delineated. All of our lives come back to them in our daydreams..." Gaston Bachelard

Believing in what Bachelard said, I am jotting in some information about the houses from which our homes have evolved so you children and grandchildren may have a stimulus to recall the cellars, garrets, nooks and crannies, etc., of your past at our homes.

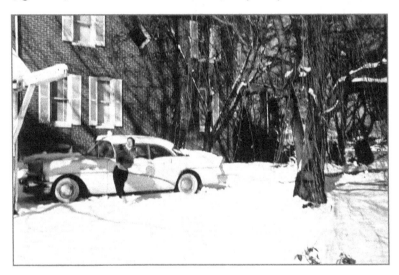

FIG 16-A: Our first apartment after marriage in 1957. On Rosemont Ave, in Frederick, MD (Jeanette in snow). We arrived here from Memphis and I had bought some basic furniture from a discount sale in Frederick: a modern L-sectional couch with powder blue fabric accented with a gold thread and supported by peg-shaped exposed wooden legs; a maple-backed chair and bed frame with bookcase headboard. I had my 12 inch black and white TV from the BOQ. For the next 50 years Jeanette subtly commented on her initial reaction to her new home. It seems that late in the afternoon the couch took on a slightly fluorescent glow. Suffice to say changes were made.

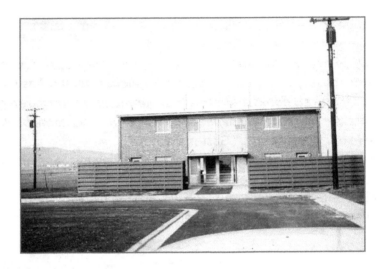

FIG. 16-B: Our second home (1958) in the new officers' quarters (right half) at Ft. Detrick, MD. This is where we lived when Carla was born. As a Captain in U. S. Army at WRAMC in Ft. Detrick we were provided beautiful new quarters for which all services were provided.

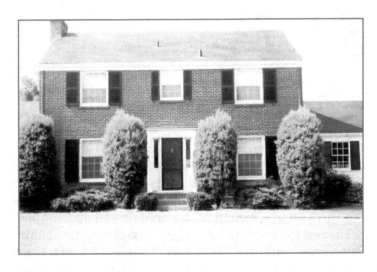

FIG. 16-C: The first house we bought on Chadwick Road, in Moorgate Subdivision in Louisville, for the enormous price of $26,000 (before the Jeanette-Walter touch).

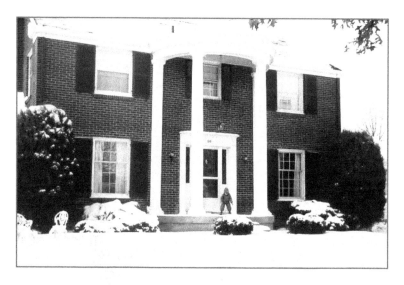

FIG. 16-D: Same house as FIG. 16-C after Jeanette-Walter touch. Carla on front porch.

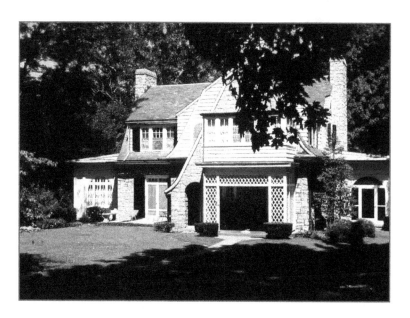

FIG. 16-E: The second home we bought; on 1556 Cherokee Rd, Louisville, 40205; from the back yard; the front overlooked Cherokee Park. This is where we lived when Chris was born.

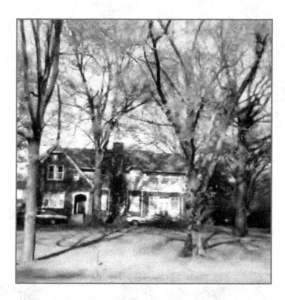

FIG. 16-F: Our first house in Memphis after move from Louisville in 1969. Located at 578 Center Drive in Hein Park, adjacent to Rhodes College campus and Overton Park (where Jeanette and I had our first date). We added a den to the back, repainted inside and out, re-landscaped and Jeanette decorated the entire house. After 3 years realtors begged us to sell to an interested client. We were not interested; we liked this place; they persisted; finally to end the plight, I mentioned a sale price more than double our investment. Surprisingly, it was accepted and a delightful young 20+ year old member of a rock music group and recipient of an Academy Award, wrote a check for payment-in-full, with less stress than Jeanette and I had in making our monthly mortgage payment. We were fortunate to find another "jewel".

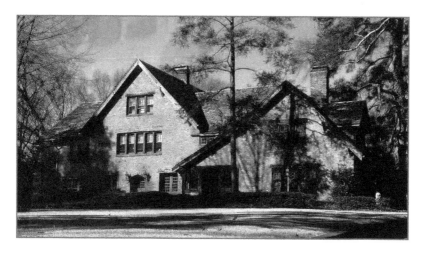

Fig. 16-G: Our second house in Memphis; a 7,000 sq. ft. classic English Tudor with slate roof on two acres at 3438 Central Ave. with tennis court, garage apartment and many leaves to rake. We moved from this house to Baltimore.

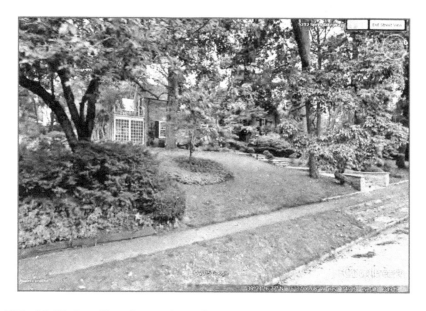

FIG. 16-H: Our first home in Baltimore at 5212 Springlake Way, Homeland overlooking small lakes.

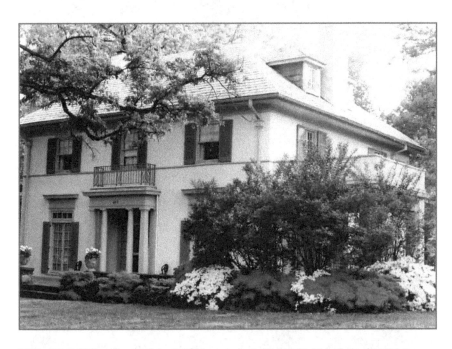

FIG. 16-I: Our second in Baltimore at 4312 St. Paul St., 21210; near Homewood Campus at Johns Hopkins University; after stucco repair by Walter, exterior paint by Greg and Chris and Interior decoration by Jeanette.

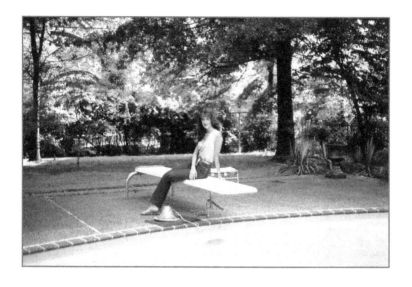

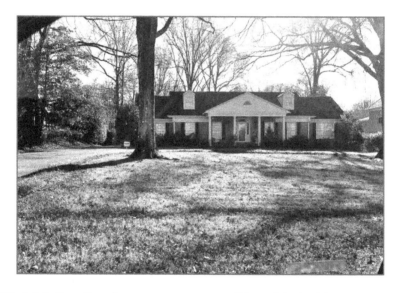

FIG. 16-J: Our first house on return to Memphis in 1981 at 3733 S. Galloway Dr., 38111 on Galloway Golf Course. Carla (Shown) and Greg are at U. of Memphis and Chris is at home.

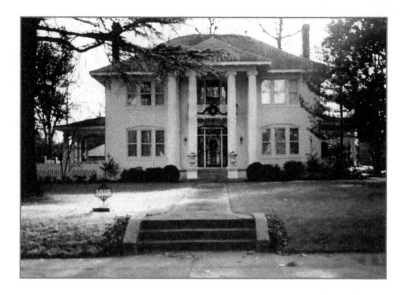

FIG. 16-K: Our second house after return from Baltimore on 1615 Central Ave. in Memphis, 38111. We undertook major restoration, added a garage and a brick patio (with Chris's help).

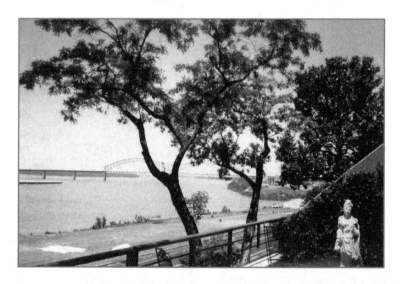

FIG. 16-L: Our downsize as empty nesters, a two bedroom condominium at 385 Chickasaw Bluff, Memphis 38103, overlooking the Mighty Mississippi River. This is where we lived when Carla was married.

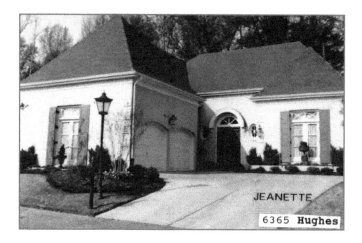

FIG. 16-M: Back to traditional out east family house with room for grandchildren on 6365 Winfrey Place, 38119.

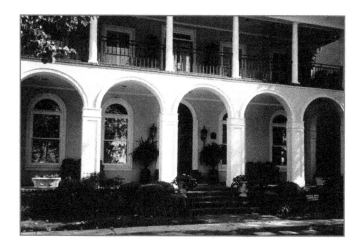

FIG. 16-N: Eureka!! This is it. 854 River Park Drive in Harbor Town on Mud Island in the Mississippi River. We bought it in 1993 and never moved again. Once we moved to this new house built by Greer Collins, Jeanette and I set out to decorate, enhance architecturally and extensively landscape the property. We were among "pioneers" taking a chance on a residential area on an island under development on the Mississippi River. Many friends questioned our sanity. Fortunately, over our 22 years here the island has become prime real estate in Memphis.

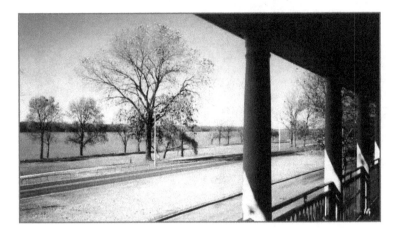

FIG. 16-O: 854 River Park Dr., view from front balcony. Jeanette loved this sight – watching the river with barges and beautiful western sunsets, children and families in Greenbelt Park, bikers, parade of pets, birds in her nearby trees and family on the balcony. She could also see this view from her bedroom window where she spent her later years enjoying her home on the river.

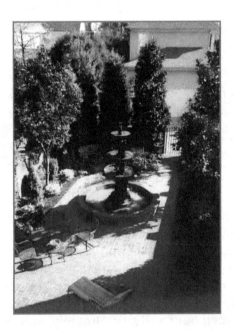

FIG. 16-P: 854 River Park Dr., east backyard garden.

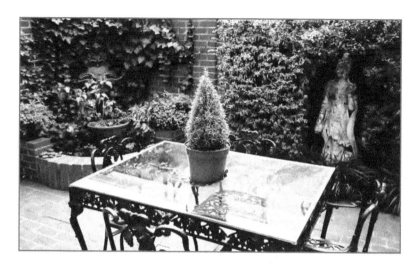

FIG. 16-Q: 854 River Park Dr., patio from den.

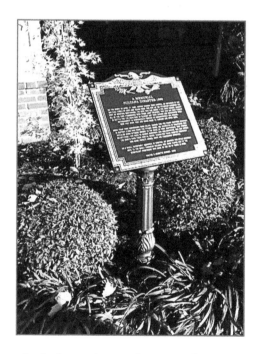

FIG. 16-R: Historical plaque in our front yard: "SULTANA DISASTER – 1865"

"ON THE NIGHT OF APRL 27, 1865, BEFORE HARBOR TOWN EXISTED, AN EXPLOSION OF THE *SULTANA* COULD BE SEEN AND HEARD FROM THIS SITE AS THE STEAMSHIP DEPARTED THE PORT OF MEMPHIS NORTHWARD. THE CIVIL WAR HAD ENDED A FEW DAYS EARLIER. ALMOST ALL OF THE 2400 PASSENGERS WERE UNION ARMY SOLDIERS. THEY HAD NOT ONLY FOUGHT IN BATTLE FOR THE ABOLUTION OF SLAVERY BUT WERE MAIMED AND DEBILITATED FROM IMPRISONMENT IN CONFEDERATE PRISONS AT ANDERSONVILLE AND CAHABA. NOW THEY WERE FREE AND GOING HOME TO FAMILIES AND LOVED ONES.

MORE THAN 1585 PASSENGERS WERE KILLED, MAKING THIS THE WORST MARITIME DISASTER IN HISTORY (1522 DIED WHEN THE *TITANIC* SANK). THE CHARACTER OF MEMPHIANS WAS REVEALED WHEN CITIZENS RUSHED TO THE RIVER AS FIRST RESPONDERS. THEY WORKED RELENTLESSLY FOR DAYS TO RESCUE SURVIVORS AND NON-SURVIVORS, WHO HAD WTHIN THE MONTH BEEN THEIR MORTAL ENEMY. CASUALTIES FILLED MEMPHIS HOSPITALS AND MANY PRIVATE HOMES. SOME 800 PASSENGERS SURVIVED.

AS A SMALL RIVERFRONT MEMORIAL IN MEMPHIS, WE DEDICATE OUR LITTLE GARDENS HERE TO THE GREAT AMERICAN SOLDIERS WHO FREED SLAVES AND TO THE BENEVOLENT MEMPHIANS WHO CAME TO THE AID OF THOSE IN NEED."

WALTER & JEANETTE HUGHES - 2013

CHAPTER 17

Pneumocystis and the Rest of the Story

Serendipity rides again!! On January 1, 1981 I came back to St. Jude and was faced with the chore of starting an entirely new program in Infectious Diseases and recruiting new faculty and fellows. I had specific plans clearly in mind in which *Pneumocystis* was relatively low priority. Surprise! I should have learned by now not to plan more than a month ahead. Earlier I had committed to some speaking engagements which I honored and here begins **"the rest of the *Pneumocystis* story."**

In April 1981 I was giving a Grand Rounds talk at the University of Pittsburgh Medical Center. As I finished a secretary in the back of the auditorium was waving one of those pink phone call slips. She informed me that I had received an urgent call from Dr. Jeffry Green in New York and that I should return it immediately; which I did. Dr. Green was a Fellow in Infectious Diseases with Dr. Henry Masur's group at New York University and was requesting my help with one of his patients, a 35 year old man who had been admitted a week earlier with PCP. He was started on TMP-SMZ in therapeutic doses and was responding well until the day of his call when the patient experienced a florid maculopapular rash and precipitous drop in the neutrophil count.

Dr. Green's question was could these events be related to TMP-SMZ? The answer was yes, because both the rash and neutropenia have been reported as adverse effects to sulfonamides. What to do was the next question. We suggested stopping TMP-SMZ and completing treatment with pentamidine isethionate. He agreed. In closing our phone call I said, "Let me know how your patient does." I always say that but no one ever does – unless I have been wrong, then I hear back.

Surprisingly, a few weeks later I received a nice letter from Dr. Green. He had given in detail the outcome of his patient. The rash resolved, the neutrophil count returned to normal, the pneumonitis cleared and the patient was discharged. An interesting part of his letter stated that he and his colleagues in New York had now seen five patients in recent months with PCP and without any discernable underlying disease. The only features in common were that the cases were all men and all were homosexual men. As a matter of historical interest I have shown a part of his letter in **(FIG.17-A)** where he comments, "We believe on the basis of our recent experience that the homosexual population is experiencing a heretofore unrecognized **Acquired Immunodeficiency**." The letter was dated May 11, 1981 and signed by Dr. Jeffry Green, Fellow in Infectious Diseases, at NYU.

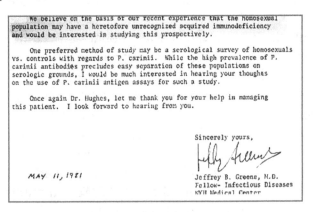

FIG. 17-A: Letter from Dr. Jeffrey Green.

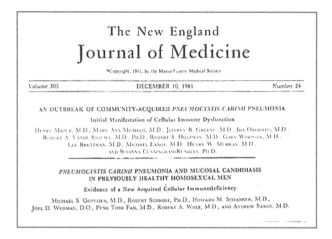

The New England
Journal of Medicine

©Copyright, 1981, by the Massachusetts Medical Society

| Volume 305 | DECEMBER 10, 1981 | Number 24 |

AN OUTBREAK OF COMMUNITY-ACQUIRED *PNEUMOCYSTIS CARINII* PNEUMONIA

Initial Manifestation of Cellular Immune Dysfunction

HENRY MASUR, M.D., MARY ANN MICHELIS, M.D., JEFFREY B. GREENE, M.D., IDA ONORATO, M.D.,
ROBERT A. VANDE STOUWE, M.D., PH.D., ROBERT S. HOLZMAN, M.D., GARY WORMSER, M.D.,
LEE BRETTMAN, M.D., MICHAEL LANGE, M.D., HENRY W. MURRAY, M.D.,
AND SUSANNA CUNNINGHAM-RUNDLES, PH.D.

PNEUMOCYSTIS CARINII PNEUMONIA AND MUCOSAL CANDIDIASIS
IN PREVIOUSLY HEALTHY HOMOSEXUAL MEN

Evidence of a New Acquired Cellular Immunodeficiency

MICHAEL S. GOTTLIEB, M.D., ROBERT SCHROFF, PH.D., HOWARD M. SCHANKER, M.D.,
JOEL D. WEISMAN, D.O., PENG THIM FAN, M.D., ROBERT A. WOLF, M.D., AND ANDREW SAXON, M.D.

FIG. 17-B: Report of first cases of AIDS, 1981.

By the end of the year in December 1981, two companion articles appeared in the **New England Journal of Medicine (FIG. 17-B)**. One article was from New York by **Dr. Henry Masur** and colleagues, including **Dr. Jeffry Green**, entitled "Community Acquired *P. carinii* Pneumonia: An Initial Manifestation of Cellular Immune Dysfunction". Their report was of 11 homosexual men with PCP and unexplained immunodeficiency. Simultaneously, **Dr. Michael Gottlieb** and colleagues in California made similar observations in homosexual men.

I mention these reports for two reasons: one is to point out that in a sense, *P. carinii* discovered AIDS. Human immunodeficiency virus (HIV) is silent and causes no discernible disease, at least early on. HIV causes immunodeficiency and the immunodeficiency allows the victim to acquire infections that are symptomatic and recognizable. Thus, when these patients with PCP came to the clinic smart doctors like Henry Masur, Jeffrey Green, Michael Gottlieb and their colleagues began to immediately search for an underlying immunocompromising disease because they knew one was always present with PCP. When no cause was found, their inquisitive minds began to search further.

A second point to make about the New York cases is that, even with the infinite beginning sample of 11 cases of AIDS, the high rate of adverse effects to TMP-SMZ became apparent in Dr. Jeffrey Green's case referred to above. Soon after these two articles several reports began to appear where very high rates of rash, neutropenia, fever, and other adverse effects occurred in HIV-infected individuals given TMP-SMZ. These rates greatly exceeded the less than 6 % seen in non-AIDS patients, reaching 20 to 50 % in some instances.

Because it soon became apparent the AIDS epidemic was gaining legs, that PCP was the cause of death in some 75% of cases, and because TMP-SMZ was in trouble for a very important role in the management of this disease, I decided to resume work on drug development for PCP treatment and prophylaxis.

By this time **Dr. Linda Pilfer** and **Dianne Wood** in our lab at St Jude had propagated *P. carinii* in embryonic chick epithelial lung cell culture, providing an *in vitro* method for drug testing. However, we did not know how predictable these methods might be in determining efficacy in human disease. On the other hand, we had clearly **validated** the corticosteroid-treated rat model for this purpose by doing a study in the rat and later repeating the same study in humans and finding the results were similar. Therefore, we chose the animal model in further studies.

During the next 10 to 12 years or so, some three grant cycles, we identified the following compounds and drugs as having very high activity against *P. carinii*. We referred to these as zero drugs because *P carinii* was found in none of the animals after a six-week course of corticosteroid immunosuppression while receiving the test compound:

1984: Diaminodiphenylsulfone **(DAPSONE)**
1986: Sulfonylurea compounds
       4, 4' sulfonylbisformaldehyde
1990: 1, 4 hydroxynaphthoquinone **(566C80 – ATOVAQUONE)**
1991: Synergy – macrolide + sulfa
1993: PS-15 (new biguanide)

1996: Mono-sulfonamides
1997: Mycophenolate mofetil
Lasalocid

We chose to take two of these drugs into clinical trials. The first was dapsone because of its early discovery and the urgent need for a new anti-PCP drug and later the 566C80 compound. I'll not comment further on the other drugs. The published references are included in **APPENDIX 1.** Several of these other drugs are excellent prospects for clinical development.

Dapsone (diaminodiphenlysulfone) is an old drug that has been in clinical use for the treatment of leprosy for more than half a century. It also has some activity against malaria. You may have realized by now that a guide we have often followed in the search for anti-*P. carinii* drugs is based on the premise that *Pneumocystis and Plasmodium sp.* tend to have similar susceptibility patterns. Fortunately, the observation by others in recent years that *P. carinii* is a fungus and not a protozoan came after we had found these drugs were effective against *P. carinii* and that the antifungal drugs were not effective.

Our animal studies showed dapsone to be as effective as TMP-SMZ in the prevention of PCP when administered orally as a single dose daily, weekly, and even monthly. It was also found to be effective therapeutically, especially when given in combination with trimethoprim. Trimethoprim had a synergistic effect with dapsone, as it did with sulfamethoxazole. Trimethoprim alone has no discernible effect on *P. carinii*. Furthermore, the trimethoprim component of TMP-SMZ is less likely to be associated with adverse effects than is the sulfonamide.

I'll not go through the clinical trials evaluating dapsone and dapsone-trimethoprim in patients with HIV infection, because they are referenced in the **APPENDIX 1.** Most of the studies were done at the University of California, San Francisco because we no longer had patients with PCP at St. Jude due to use of TMP-SMZ prophylaxis. Essentially, all the clinical studies confirmed precisely the results from animal studies and showed that dapsone and TMP-dapsone were comparable to TMP-SMZ as to efficacy in the prevention and treatment of PCP in AIDS patients, while the former had significantly fewer adverse events. Also, because of the long half-life of dapsone, we found it could be used as a one dose per week for PCP prophylaxis in patients with AIDS **APPENDIX 1**.

The pivotal randomized controlled study comparing TMP-dapsone and TMP-SMZ in the treatment of PCP in 60 AIDS patients is summarized in **(FIG. 17-C).** While the drugs were equally effective, 17 of 30 patients receiving TMP-SMZ had significant adverse effects compared to only 9 0f 30 taking TMP-Dapsone. In fact, it was found that two-thirds of AIDS patients experiencing adverse reactions to TMP-SMZ would be able to safely take TMP-dapsone. So, dapsone became a useful part of the armamentarium for the treatment and prevention of PCP.

Oral Therapy for *Pneumocystis carinii* Pneumonia in the Acquired Immunodeficiency Syndrome: a Controlled Trial of Trimethoprim-Sulfamethoxazole *versus* Trimethoprim-Dapsone

Medina I, Mills J, Leoung G, Hopewell PC, Lee B, Modin G, Benowitz N, Wofsy C, *et al.*
N Engl J Med 323: 776, 1990

	No. Patients	Treatment failure	Severe toxicity
TMP-Dapsone	30	2	9
TMP-SMZ	30	3	17

FIG. 17-C: Comparison of dapsone and SMZ with TMP in AIDS patients.

In 1988 I received a call from Dr. Win Gutteridge, Director of Parasitic Disease Drug Research, at the Wellcome Research Laboratories in Beckenham, UK. He informed me he had a new antimalarial drug still in laboratory studies that showed promise against a variety of Plasmodium species resistant to current drugs and asked if I would be interested in testing it in our animal model for activity against *P. carinii*. After hearing the compound was a 1, 4' hydroxynaphthoquinone with a mechanism of action different to the other anti-PCP drugs, I indicated I was interested. As the AIDS epidemic was rapidly expanding and use of TMP-SMZ being used worldwide for long periods of time we expected that eventually resistance to the antifol drugs would occur. So, I suggested that Dr. Gutteridge send me an aliquot of the compound and I would add it to one of our animal studies. However, the compound was still a powder in a bottle, so dosage, route of administration, absorption and pharmacokinetics would need to be worked out for our rat model.

Soon thereafter, Dr. Vicki Latter from Guttridge's group arrived at my office at St. Jude in Memphis with a supply of their new compound #566C80, in her purse. A remarkably bright and capable Microbiologist, Dr. Latter spent a few days in our lab telling us about 566C80 and learning about our animal model and *P. carinii,* an organism that had not been a focus of their research.

A background story of historical interest was that under new global leadership the Burroughs-Wellcome Co. was considering the termination of their Parasitic Disease Drug Branch, in part because the company had for decades continually lost extensive finances in developing and providing antiparasitic drugs. A current question before the administration was whether or not to undertake further development of #566C80, despite early evidence as a promising antimalarial drug. A consultant parasitologist from Gaithersburg, MD, Dr. Craig Canfield, pointed out that if the new compound also had activity against other diseases, it perhaps might be worth pursuing further. He suggested Dr.Gutteridge contact me about testing the compound for anti-*P carinii* activity in our animal model. This led to my introduction to the saga.

Soon after Vicki left we began a screening study to hopefully learn whether or not #566C80 had anti-*P. carinii* activity.

It is at this point in time that I began my story on page 1, Chapter 1 of this book. I was scheduled to give a presentation at the annual meeting of the Society of Parasitologists on July 20, 1988 in

Bristol, England. We had begun the 566C80 animal studies on June 1, 1988, so I expected to have some preliminary data at the time of the Bristol meeting. Plans were made to meet privately with Win Gutteridge and colleagues who would also be attending the meeting. Members and speakers of the Society were to be housed in the ancient dormitory rooms at the University of Bristol – a macho thing from the planning committee, so the Wellcome group decided to meet with me in the more luxurious Lounge of the Bristol Hotel.

I spent the full day before I left for England reading the coded lung biopsy slides from our study and barely finished in time to get from the lab at St. Jude to the Memphis Airport. With results from my reading of blind-coded slides jotted in pencil on a yellow legal pad plus the sealed protocol code that had been held by the Pharmacist, stuffed in my briefcase, I spent much of the time over the Atlantic decoding and tabulating results.

At precisely 6:00 pm some 5 or 6 folk from Wellcome and I seated ourselves around a cocktail table in the Bristol Hotel Lounge. After a brief chitchat and my sense that expectations were low among the group, I gave a five-minute summary of our experimental design and proceeded to the results, which I had tabulated in longhand on one legal pad page. The following is the total content of the page I passed around to the group:

STUDY GROUP	NO.	(%) RATS WITH PCP
CONTROL (NO DRUG)	10/10	100 %
CONTROL (TMP-SMZ)	0/8	0 %
DRUG A	10/10	100 %
DRUG B	8/9	89 %
DRUG C (#566C80)	0/10	0 % **
DRUG D	10/10	100 %
DRUG E	7/7	100 %
DRUG F	9/10	90 %
DRUG G	10/10	100 %
DRUG H	8/8	100 %
DRUG I	7/7	100%

The results showed clearly that #566C80 is effective against *P. carinii* pneumonitis in the animal model in that **none** of the rats given #566C80 during six weeks of corticosteroid immunosuppression acquired PCP while **all** of those not given the drug had PCP at autopsy. Conversation rose to a higher, louder and more joyful level for the remainder of the evening while some scattered to make phone calls.

After completion of our initial animal studies, the Wellcome group repeated them in Beckenham, UK and found similar results. Overall, the animal studies showed #566C80 to be as effective as TMP-SMZ in the prevention of PCP when administered orally as a single dose daily, three-days a week or once every two weeks. The drug was also as effective as TMP-SMZ in the treatment of established PCP and response was dose related. Absorption of the compound was poor but could be enhanced by the administration of a fatty meal with doses. **APPENDIX 1**

The next issue to resolve was whether or not #566C80 should be taken to clinical trials, and if so, should it be evaluated as an antimalarial drug or an anti-PCP drug. At the time a conservative estimate for the cost of development to FDA approval was about 250 million dollars, if all went well. After several meetings among Burroughs-Wellcome-UK, Burroughs-Wellcome-USA and other planners the administrative decision was made to proceed with clinical trials of #566C80 in patients with AIDS. I was asked to serve as the Principal Investigator for the clinical trials, which I agreed to do. Perhaps my *pro bono* status for the company, accounted for my selection as much as my investigative prowess. I received salaried support from St. Jude Children's Research Hospital, as an endowed Arthur Ash Chairmanship in Pediatric AIDS Research and N. I. H. grants that allowed considerable liberty in my research – an important factor in my work for which I have always been grateful.

We knew that #566C80 was 1, 4' hydroxynaphthoquinone, an analogue of ubiquinone (vitamin K) and that similar drugs were usually of low toxicity. The mechanism of action as determined in *Plasmodium,* species was inhibition of mitochondrial respiration and electron transport by binding *dihydroorotate dehydrogenase* at cytochrome bc$_1$ (Complex III).

The first clinical trial was done at St. Jude Children's Research in 1990-91. The Phase 1 Study enrolled 19 HIV-infected men recruited with the help of our colleagues in the Department of Medicine at the University of Tennessee College of Medicine.

At this time in mid-America AIDS still harbored fear among lay public, despite sound scientific knowledge that provided us safety from transmission with proper precautions. The early opposition to AIDS research at St. Jude is discussed elsewhere in this book but I must make a special point here to recognize some noble people related to this study. First is appreciation for the brave and dedicated 19 grown men with HIV infection who came to a children's hospital, via a back door after the day clinics had closed, took a chemical compound with the understanding that it might cause them harm and under the design of the current study would provide them no benefit, underwent tests and repeated observations and demanded nothing in return except the satisfaction of having been of some help to their fellow man.

Phase 1 studies are difficult to do because of the need for precision in drug administration, blood sampling and clinical observations. Key to this effort was our superb Nurse Practitioner, Wren Kennedy with the support of her colleagues Glenda Fullen, Debra Rosenbaum and others listed in the authorship of the study. I was required to seek waivers for a few institutional policies to admit adult homosexual men with HIV to the children's hospital for a phase 1 study, etc. Detailed precautions were developed. Despite some unrest among his faculty the Director of St. Jude at the time, Dr. Joe Simone, granted approval as well as positive support for our studies.

The results of the Phase 1 Study in HIV-infected men are shown in **(FIG. 17-D)**. The only adverse event was a mild rash in one patient that cleared while still on the drug; furthermore, the plasma half-life of 51 hours was an added advantage.

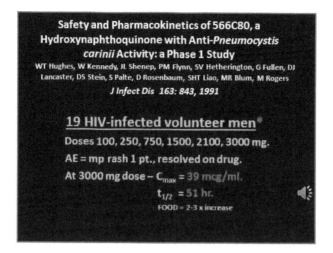

FIG. 17-D: Results of the first clinical trial, a Phase 1 study of safety and pharmacokinetics of #566C80.

The next step was a preliminary study to evaluate #566C80 as to therapeutic efficacy. Because we no longer had PCP cases at St. Jude, a multicenter study was established to include investigators at the University of Tennessee College of Medicine; the University of Cincinnati Medical Center; the Clinical Center at the National Institutes of Health, Baylor University Medical Center and George Washington University. Thirty-four patients with AIDS and PCP were treated with #566C80, now given the generic name of Atovaquone. The results shown in **(FIG. 17-E)** revealed the drug to offer promise as to efficacy and safety.

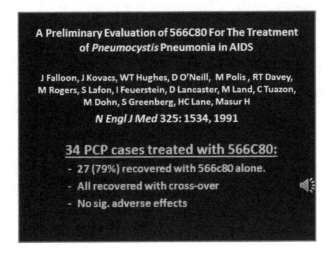

FIG. 17-E: 79 % of PCP patients recovered with #566C80 alone and there were no significant adverse effects.

A pivotal study required by the FDA was a comparison of Atovaquone with the standard for treatment, TMP-SMZ. Statisticians informed us that at least 300 HIV-infected patients with PCP would be required to determine if Atovaquone was no less effective than TMP-SMZ. This was a rather staggering number because of the diminishing number of PCP cases available for study. To power the study to determine if Atovoquone was superior to TMP-SMZ would be prohibitive. A large multicenter double blind, randomized study was organized to include 52 clinical centers throughout the United States as well as Canada, Puerto Rico and Europe. Enrollment of 322 patients was accomplished in a reasonable period of time and the results are displayed in **(FIG. 17-F)**.

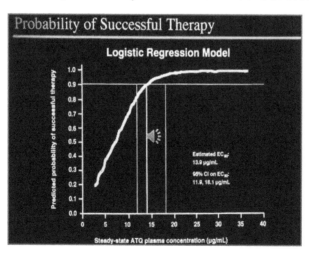

Comparison of Atovaquone (566C80) with Trimethoprim-Sulfamethoxazole to Treat *P. carinii* Pneumonia in Patients with AIDS

Walter Hughes, Gifford Leoung, Francoise Kramer, Samuel Bozzette, Sharon Safron, Peter Frame, Nathan Clumeck, Henry Masur, Danny Lancaster, Charles Chan, James Lavelle, Joel Rosenstock, Judith Falloon, Judith Feinberg, Stephen LaFon, Michael Rogers, Fred Sattler & NIH-ACTG*

N Engl J Med 328: 1521, 1993

Drug	No. Patients	Efficacy Failure	T-L Adverse Event	Therapy Success
ATOVAQUONE	160	20%	7%	62%
TMP-SMZ	162	7%	20%	64%

FIG. 17-F: The protocol-driven definitions of therapeutic success showed the drugs to be similar. This was because of better safety with atovaquone and better efficacy of TMP-SMZ.

We compared the steady-state atovaquone plasma concentration values with the therapeutic success rates and found therapeutic success was directly related to plasma concentrations of atovaquone.

FIG. 17-G: Relationship of steady-state plasma concentration and therapeutic success.

All of the animal and human trials to this point in time were done using a tablet formulation of atovaquone. Our pharmacokinetic and other studies showed poor and somewhat erratic absorption. A new liquid formulation was developed by Burroughs-Wellcome, which is now the formulation of choice.

The following is a summary of the Atovaquone studies, going from compound on the shelf to FDA approval in less than 6 years:

- 1990: Animal studies—effective prophylaxis and treatment.
- 1991: Phase 1 studies – safety and pharmacokinetics I man.
- 1992: Preliminary trial – effective treatment
- 1994: Comparison of atovaquone and TMP-SMZ in treatment of PCP
- 1994: FDA approval (Mepron[R])

ESTIMATE OF USAGE AND IMPACT OF ST. JUDE anti-PCP DRUGS:

It is not possible to give a precise account of the total usage of TMP-SMZ, dapsone and atovaquone for the treatment and prevention of PCP since the original introduction of TMP-SMZ in 1977 because of generic designations, multiple manufacturers worldwide, change in brand names, etc. However, the following information gives a reasonable grasp of usage under certain circumstances.

<u>**Recommendations in textbooks and guidelines:**</u> TMP-SMZ has been unchallenged as the drug of choice recommended for the treatment and prevention of PCP for more than 35 years. Prophylaxis is recommended for high-risk patients with cancer, congenital immunodeficiency disorders, organ transplant recipients and AIDS.

Recommendations from the Centers for Disease Control (CDC), Infectious Diseases Society of America (IDSA), National Institutes of Health (NIH) 1989 to present time: In 1989 an expert committee (of which I was a member) from the CDC, IDSA and NIH instituted federally supported guidelines for the management of opportunistic infections in HIV-infected patients. These guidelines have been continually updated since inception and have become the physician's "bible" in management of HIV/AIDS **(FIG. 17-H)**.

- TMP-SMZ HAS BEEN RECOMMENDED AS THE DRUG OF CHOICE FOR THE TREATMENT AND PREVENTION OF PATIENTS WITH HIV/AIDS SINCE 1989.

- THE CURRENT RECOMMENDATION IS AS FOLLOWS FOR PROPHYLAXIS:

Give TMP-SMZ daily, or three days a week, as PCP prophylaxis for all HIV-infected patients while the CD^4 T lymphocyte counts less than 200 cells/mm^3

Alternative drugs recommended: dapsone, atovaquone and aerosol pentamidine.

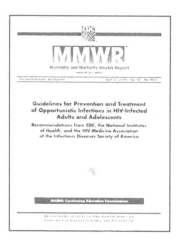

FIG. 17-H: MMWR PUBLICATION OF CDC, NIH AND IDSA GUIDELINES.

ESTIMATION OF USAGE OF ST JUDE DRUGS FOR PREVENTION OF PCP IN HIV/AIDS 2012:

A recent study provides information that allows us to roughly calculate the global use of PC prophylaxis in HIV/AIDS patients. The TAHO database from 19 global sites published in the **Journal of International AIDS Society, 15:1, 2012** determined the number of HIV/AIDS patients eligible for PCP prophylaxis by the CDC, IDSA, NIH and WHO guidelines. Furthermore, the study also determined the number of HIV/AIDS patients who are actually taking anti-PCP drugs. Using WHO Reports of the total number of HIV/AIDS now living in the world, we are able to estimate the usage of St Jude drugs (TMP-SMZ, dapsone and atovaquone) as follows:

- **HIV/AIDS patients eligible for PCP prophylaxis = 20 %**
- **HIV/AIDS patients receiving PCP prophylaxis = 14 %**
- **No. People living with HIV/AIDS: WHO Report, 2011**
  - **Worldwide = 32.2 million**
  - **USA = 1.0 million**

THUS, WORLDWIDE SOME 4.8 MILLION PATIENTS WITH HIV/AIDS ARE CURRENTLY RECEIVING ST JUDE ANTI-PCP DRUGS AND ABOUT 140,000 OF THESE ARE IN THE USA.

These figures do not include the St. Jude anti-PCP drugs used to treat PCP in AIDS patients. Also, they do not include the use of drugs for the prevention of treatment of patients with cancer, congenital immunodeficiency disorders and organ transplant recipients.

CHAPTER 18

St. Jude and AIDS

I ask you to think back again to January, 1981 when I returned to St. Jude, so I can tell you about aspects of our work beyond that just described in chapter 17 for *Pneumocystis carinii.*

Coming back to our offices and labs on the fourth floor of ALSAC Tower was nostalgic, but lonely, and it was a cold winter in January. Most of the group I had accrued had departed, so I was in a sense starting over. As at Hopkins in 1977, I now had offices and labs to fill with faculty and fellows.

Be aware at this time the Acquired Immunodeficiency Syndrome (AIDS) was still in the process of being discovered. My unique pre-view in April and May 1981 is described in chapter 17, but it was not until December 1981 that the definitive reports of Masur, *et al* and Gottlieb, *et al,* as well as others appeared. I mention this to point out that I had in no way planned for research in AIDS beyond drugs for PCP. In fact nothing could be further from a rational area for research at St. Jude Children's Research Hospital in the early 1980s than AIDS. At that time it was a mysterious entity occurring in sexually active ho-mosexual men and adult iv drug addicts in New York and California; the cause was unknown but it resulted in a wipeout of the immune system and 100 % fatality from opportunistic infections.

Because *Pneumocystis carinii* pneumonia (PCP) was the cause of death in at least 70 % of AIDS cases and I was one of only a few physician-scientists with considerable experience in the field, I became involved nationally as a consultant, seminar speaker, member of governmental and non-governmental Committees in the adult world of AIDS. This was not a Pediatric disease. As the AIDS epidemic spread PCP rapidly evolved from an obscure opportunistic infection to one of global importance and we focused on the pneumonitis, but not AIDS.

In **1981** recruitment went briskly and I was especially fortunate to bring **Jerry L. Shenep, MD** from Washington University in St. Louis where he finished a Fellowship in Infectious Diseases. His work on the lipopolysaccharides of *Haemophilus influenza* provided a sound base for similar studies with Gram-negative bacilli common to the immunocompromised host. Also, my old colleague **Sandor Feldman, MD** responded to the St. Jude homing device and returned to resume his studies on varicella-zoster virus infections, a major hazard to immunosuppressed children with cancer. In 1982 **Dennis Stokes, MD,** my colleague at Hopkins, was recruited to head the Cardiopulmonary Intensive Unit, founded by Dr. Sam Sanyal, at St. Jude and placed in our department because of common research and clinical interests.

In **1982-83** we added **John W. Sixbey, MD**, an Internist and Infectious Diseases Specialist from the University of North Carolina at Chapel Hill who was undertaking interesting research with Epstein-Barr virus infections and **Francis Gigliotti, MD** a dynamic physician-scientist in Pediatric Infectious Diseases from the University of Rochester in New York who would develop monoclonal antibodies for diagnostic and therapeutic uses.

A close affiliation was established with the new Division of Infectious Diseases, Department of Pediatrics at the University of Tennessee College of Medicine and Le Bonheur Children's Hospital under the directorship of **Fred Barrett, MD,** an established national leader in Pediatric Infectious diseases from Baylor College of Medicine and one who would become a life-long friend. This important relationship provided a sound basis for fellowship training in Pediatric Infectious Diseases combing research (St. Jude) and clinical (Le Bonheur) experiences._

1984-85 was a busy year. Dr. Joe Simone had become the Director of St. Jude, the position previously held by Dr. Alvin Mauer and Dr. Donald Pinkel. The institution was growing in all dimensions. The annual budget was now $38,786,617. My role was moved up a notch to a new position of **Chairman of Child Health Sciences** which encompassed all of the rapidly growing non-oncology clinical research and service units at St. Jude. The intent was to have combined productive research programs with essential services to provide optimal patient management. We organized it as the following **Divisions** (with Directors): **Infectious Diseases** (Walter Hughes, MD); **Cardiopulmonary Diseases** (Dennis Stokes, MD); **Nutrition and Metabolism** (Paulus Zee, PhD, MD); **Dentistry** (Kenneth Hopkins, DDS); **Psychiatry** (Abby L. Wasserman, MD); **Psychology** (Raymond K. Mulhern, PhD); **Neurology** (Edward Kovnar, MD); **Comparative Medicine and Animal Science** (Jerold E. Rehg, DVM); and Hospital **Infection Control** (Bobby Williams, EHT).

"Yes! Here we go again, you just couldn't say no. Why couldn't someone else do all that?" Jeanette said. Somewhere along the way, I don't recall exactly when, the **Nursing Division** was under my administrative domain. It was here I came to appreciate the **Nurse,** in particular the **St. Jude Nurse.** All doctors should spend time in the shoes of nurses before being allowed to practice medicine. I subsequently followed Jeanette's philosophy to do "what **you** think is right and best."

On **April 16, 1984** Danny Thomas received the Congressional Gold Medal, the highest civilian award given by the U. S Congress for his humanitarian efforts on behalf of St. Jude Children's' Research Hospital. President Ronald Regan made the presentation.

In 1984 we established <u>The John H. Erskine Lectureship</u> at St. Jude in honor of the medical officer of the Memphis Health Department who gave his life in the service of his patients during the 1878 Yellow Fever epidemic. Dr. John Sixbey told me of his historical research on Erskine. I was impressed and asked Joe Simone to support the annual lectureship that he approved. Now, some three decades later the lecture has been delivered annually by icons in infectious diseases and Nobel Award recipients*: 1984- Theodore Woodward, MD.,

U. Maryland; 1985- Anthony S. Fauci, MD, NIH; 1986- D. Carleton Gajdusek*, MD, NIH; 1987- Saul Krugman, MD, New York U.; 1988- M. A. Epstein, CBE, FRS, U Oxford; 1989- Jonas E.Salk, MD, PhD, Salk Institute; 1990- George Klein, MD, Karolinska Institute; 1991-Tomsiaku Kawasaki, MD, Kawasaki Research Center; 1992- Baruch Blumberg*, MD, PhD, Fox Chase Cancer Center; 1994- Samuel L. Katz, MD, Duke U.; 1995- David A. Kessler, MD, FDA; 1996- Stanley B. Prusner*,MD, U. Calif.; 1997- David Ho, MD, Aaron Diamond AIDS Research Center.

Now, loyal readers and relatives I am going to tell you the true story of a St. Jude patient. My words are not adequate to relate the significance of this story. What follows is not fictional but indeed a factual account of the patient that had an influence on St. Jude, as well as others and myself. Of course, to protect the identity of our patient I have substituted all identifiers.

In 1986 "Jane Doe", a young St. Jude patient who had successfully completed two and half years of chemotherapy and was cured of acute lymphocytic leukemia returned to the hospital with a sudden onset of fever, diffuse pneumonia, and bloodstream infection due to *Streptococcus pneumoniae*. The leukemia was still in complete remission. A lung biopsy revealed lymphoid interstitial pneumonia and an ELISA for HTLV-3 (old term for HIV) antigen was positive. She now had AIDS from exchange blood transfusions she had received earlier to survive leukemia. Now the sad saga begins.

In 1986 the diagnosis of AIDS carried a profound stigma and fear that ostracized victims from society. In contrast to the cure of leukemia, AIDS was universally fatal; no one survived and most patients were dead within two years. These patients were like lepers of old; no one would touch them. Only one drug Azidothymidine (AZT) was known to have some temporary effects on AIDS in adults but had not been tested in or approved for children. By conventional practice one would send the patient home for maximal comfort and supportive care for a peaceful demise; death was certain. However, some St. Jude doctors took the "old St. Jude stance" and set out to get some AZT and treat her, others were opposed. Nevertheless, we learned that an AIDS Clinical Trial Group (ACTG) from the National

Institutes of Health was opening a protocol to evaluate AZT in children at Duke University, but no cases had been enrolled. We were able through St. Jude funding, to send our Jane Doe to Duke as the first enrollee and thus the first child to our knowledge to receive antiretroviral treatment for HIV infection.

Upon return to St. Jude for subsequent management, some controversy resumed. We were criticized for spending institutional funds to send her and her parents to Duke for the drug, for using ICU beds for episodic admissions, the use of doctors' and nurses' time and giving false hope to patient and family when the immediate outcome was death in 100% of cases. Here I must acknowledge stalwart support of Dr. Lois Dow (Hematology), Dr. Joe Simone (Director) and Drs. John Sixbey, Jerry Shenep, Pat Flynn and others in the Department of Infectious Diseases for the support of our stance on AIDS.

The outcome of the Jane Doe case explains why some doctors take a chance on experimental drugs and hesitate to pull the plug of a respirator. Our patient experienced recurrent episodes of pneumonia, disseminated varicella, pneumococcal sepsis, influenza and other infections that were satisfactorily treated as they arose. As AZT began to fail to control the HIV infection, new experimental drugs were becoming available for management at St. Jude as our Pediatric AIDS program evolved. She over time received didanosine, lamivudine, ritonavir, saquinavir, abacavir, efavirenz, amprenavir, kaletra, and others. Of course, trimethoprim-sulfamethoxazole prophylaxis prevented *Pneumocystis* pneumonia throughout her course.

MIRACULOUS LESSON:

MORE THAN TWENTY-FIVE YEARS AFTER DIAGNOSIS OF AIDS OUR PATIENT "Jane Doe" LIVES; SHE GRADUATED FROM HIGH SCHOOL AND WAS MARRIED IN 1998. YOU CAN DEDUCE IN YOUR OWN MINDS THE MORAL OF THIS TRUE STORY. I can't say more at this point. I'm going on to 85 years you know and don't have a lot of time; however, I expanded on a similar event in my novel, **Suffer the Little Children.**

1987 was the year of St. Jude's 25th Anniversary. At an earlier meeting of the Executive Committee Dr. Simone asked the department chairmen to submit suggestions for an entirely new research effort for St. Jude in the realm of catastrophic diseases of childhood. Plans were underway to break ground for construction of a five-story research tower and two-story parking garage adjacent to the hospital building. It was expected that by the time the building would be completed in late 1989 some 60 to 100 new scientific staff would be added, with a doubling of research expenditures. New research programs would be possible.

On **April 26, 1987** I submitted a six-page proposal entitled,

"PROPOSAL FOR THE ESTABLSHMENT OF A RESEARCH CENTER FOR PEDIATRC ACQURED IMMUNODEFICIENCY SYNDROME (AIDS) AT ST. JUDE CHILDREN'S RESEARCH HOSPTAL."

On **May 5, 1987** Dr. Simone, endorsed the first phase of my proposal, i.e., to explore the feasibility of the program at St. Jude through local and national interviews and investigations and data collection.

On **August 11, 1987** I submitted the detailed feasibility study to the Director, resulting from my interviews and presentations to the St. Jude faculty, Regional Directors of ALSAC, nurses, technicians, housekeepers, social workers and open seminars for anyone; involved faculty in the Depts. of Medicine and Pediatrics at University of Tennessee, Memphis-Shelby Co. Health Dept.; visits to other cancer centers and hospitals in the U.S. related to AIDS; and, presentation of our proposal to Dr. John R. La Montague, Director of AIDS program, National Institute of Allergy and Infectious Diseases, NIH for his opinion .

After noting expected problems and benefits I specified the details of the program that would require me to be relieved of responsibilities of the Dept. of Child Health Sciences (Jeanette liked this) and expansion of the Dept. of Infectious Diseases that would incorporate AIDS research. I would chair the department.

On **November 19, 1987** at the ground-breaking ceremonies of the new research tower, a national news release was made by

Danny Thomas announcing the establishment of a **Multidisciplinary Research Program in Pediatric AIDS. (FIG. 18-A)**

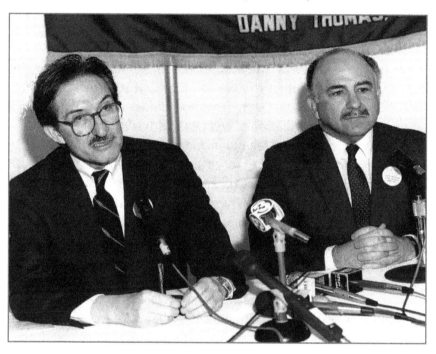

FIG. 18-A: Press conference following Danny Thomas announcement on November 19, 1987 that St. Jude was beginning a research program in Pediatric AIDS with Dr. Walter Hughes (left), the project director and Chairman, Department of Infectious Diseases and Dr. Joe Simone (right), Director of St. Jude.

The existing faculty and staff in the Department of Infectious Diseases provided a sound base for AIDS research because of our focus on infections in the immunocompromised host over the past 17 years and AIDS was essentially a syndrome of opportunistic infections.

Faculty from other Departments including Hematology/Oncology, Virology, Pharmacology, Psychology, and Immunology had indicated some interest in AIDS-related research.

Our Department and the Department of Immunology had existed side by side on the 4th floor for many years based on Dr. Don

Pinkel's intent to mix clinical researchers and basic scientists. I mention this to acknowledge Don's wisdom that resulted in a major effort to develop a polyvalent HIV vaccine by **Karen Slobod, MD** (Infectious Diseases) and **Julia Hurwitz, PhD** (Immunology) in later years of the St. Jude AIDS research endeavor. My office was adjacent to that of **Peter Doherty, PhD** with the hope that some of his brilliance might seep by osmosis through the wall to me; that part didn't work. **J. Victor Garcia, PhD** in the Dept. of Virology under took studies on cell surface CD_4 down-regulation of *Nef* gene with NIH funding.

I recruited additional faculty including **Christian C. Patrick, MD, PhD** from Baylor College of Medicine; **Seth Hetherington, MD**, from Albany University Medical Center, NY, **R. V. Srinivas, PhD** from U. Alabama and **Patricia M. Flynn, MD,** who was completing our Infectious Diseases Fellowship at St. Jude. Four research nurses and six research technicians were hired.

We initially focused on new drugs for Opportunistic infections of AIDS (see Chapter 17). **Dr. Jerry Shenep** established an essential encrypted HIV Registry for patient resources and accomplished our first anti-HIV drug study with a double blind, placebo-controlled trial of diethyldithiocarbamate in HIV-infected children and adolescents. Jerry and Pat Flynn soon rose to leadership roles in the Pediatric AIDS research efforts at both St. Jude and nationally.

We continually held that St. Jude would not serve as a treatment center, but would rather admit patients on specific protocols for research purposes only. Other resources were available for treatment of AIDS patients. Nevertheless, anxiety emerged among some employees and others at St. Jude who opposed the presence of HIV-infected people as well as any research efforts. For the most part they stayed anonymous but created unrest among some parents, some employees, some ALSAC workers, some Board members and the local news media.

While flack came from several directions the majority of doctors and nurses at St. Jude did not oppose the program and a few even openly supported it. Stalwart in support were **Dr. Joe Simone** and **Danny Thomas.** Jeanette and I, along with another St. Jude couple, were invited by Danny and Rose Marie Thomas to a private dinner party for a few friends at their home in Beverly Hills on Sept. 4, 1987. It was memorable to Jeanette sitting in the living room with celebrities of screen and TV and to me from Danny's comments in support of AIDS research at St. Jude. It was 2 months later he announced AIDS research at St. Jude.

Most of the hate messages were sent to me, Joe Simone, and indirectly to Danny. Mine were found under my office door, attached to bulletin boards, walls of elevators, in local mailboxes or in the local newspaper. The following are some examples:

"AIDS patients will spread secretions on toilet seats at St. Jude. Dr. Hughes and other doctors have private toilets."

****

"We don't want adult homosexual men with AIDS around our children at St. Jude. "Where's Danny? When homosexuals with AIDS are treated and given free run of St. Jude Children's Research Hospital - when Dr. Hughes brings drug-abusing AIDS infected mothers into the clinic - when the immunosuppressed children under treatment at St. Jude are exposed to the above - WHERE? Safe at home of course."

****

AIDS is always fatal so why treat it?

****

"We have our pity for AIDS patients who have become infected through no fault of their own. Perverted homosexual practices such as fisting and riming has led to this virus and it is **GOD'S** way of punishing both of them, and us for being so permissive...**Remember Sodom and Gomorrah."**

****

The hate notes were balanced by a few quiet accolades from friends and also from people I did not know. Some check donations began to come in from sympathetic individuals and later some came from organizations that wanted to support AIDS research. Fortunately, the local press seemed on our side with favorable publicity while publishing derogatory letters to the editor, as they should have rightly done. I recall the **Commercial Appeal** sent their science reporter to cover a presentation I made at the International Conference on AIDS in Amsterdam and wrote favorable comments for Memphians to read. The cartoon in **(FIG. 18-B)** reflects the ultimate outcome of the publicity at St. Jude.

A powerful boost to the St. Jude AIDS research program came with a $ 1,250,000 endowment initiated from an anonymous donor to establish the **ARTHUR ASHE CHAIR FOR PEDIATRIC AIDS RESEARCH**. This perhaps more than anything provided permanence to AIDS research at St. Jude. I recall the efforts of former Memphis Mayor Dick Hackett and others from ALSAC in bringing this event about. I was honored to be the first recipient of Arthur Ashe Chair. For you kids who don't know, Arthur Ashe was a famous African American tennis champion who died of AIDS a week before he was to make the presentation at the Kroger-St. Jude Tennis Classic in Memphis. He was a princely man who brought honor to his sport and race. He had received treatment with St. Jude anti PCP drugs.

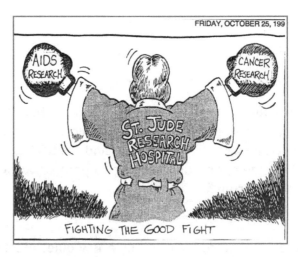

FIG. 18-B: Cartoon in Memphis Health Care News indicating support for St. Jude's new research in AIDS.

We successfully completed several clinical trials in AIDS patients at St. Jude from **1988 through 1991**. By this time I came to realize two important factors that would limit the future progress of AIDS research at St. Jude. **First**, the number of infants and children with HIV infection available to us in the mid-South was small, limiting our trials to phase 1 studies; more definitive studies could only be accomplished anywhere in the U. S. through multi-center studies. **Secondly**, the extent of St. Jude support was less secure from the Interim Director, replacing Joe Simone who left to become Physician-in-Chief at Memorial Sloan-Kettering Cancer Center in New York in 1992. It would be another year before a new Director would be on board. Also sadly, our founder and advocate **Danny Thomas** died in **1991**.

In order to move our program continually forward I decided to seek affiliation with the National Institutes of Health as a Pediatric AIDS Clinical Trials Unit (PACTU) similar to the ACTG network operating nationally for studies in adults with AIDS. The obligatory governmental regulations and bureaucracy would limit to some extent the opportunity to pursue our original ideas and experimental design we had enjoyed at St. Jude, but it would provide access to multicenter studies and financial support.

In **1992** I became the Principle Investigator of an NIAID (1- U01- A132908) grant of $3,280,634.00 to cover our PACTU from **1992- 1997** and the grant was renewed in 1997 for additional $4,507,078.00 for the next four years. Also, my NIAID-R01 grant supported our laboratory studies to discover new anti PCP drugs from 1983-1995 (total = $1,046,514.00). As the program progressed additional outside financial support came from individual faculty research grants, contributions from sympathetic supporters, grants from Pharmaceutical companies, as well as funds from St. Jude budget. A senior nucleoside pharmacologist, **Arnold Fridland, PhD,** and his colleague **Brian Robbins, PhD,** transferred from the Department of Pharmacology to Infectious Diseases, greatly enhancing our AIDS research program and NIH grant funding.

I digress for a brief explanation, lest anyone be misled. I can imagine grandchildren like Austin or Collin saying, "Gee, maybe I should be a Pediatrician like Pop, he made millions of dollars." Not so, dudes!. All those NIH grants, endowed chairs, Pharmaceutical company grants, contributions, etc. did not come to me personally. Even though I discovered the effects of TMP-SMZ, Dapsone and Atovaquone I never received a cent to the Hughes bank account. I always received a monthly paycheck based on faculty pay scale. So, if you are interested in making money talk to uncle Joe about Orthopedic Surgery or Chris about Transplant Surgeons. Pediatricians are not intended to be wealthy, but are rewarded by the happy faces of children and parents.

Early on we contributed to and benefited from the multicenter PACTG clinical trials, especially in two remarkable areas – the development of St, Jude anti PCP drugs described in Chapter 17 and the landmark PACTG Protocol 076 Study.

As the AIDS epidemic evolved "Pediatric AIDS" occurred almost exclusively as infants of HIV-infected pregnant mothers. If the transplacental passage of HIV from the infected mother to her fetus could be prevented the rapidly increasing epidemic of Pediatric AIDS would be aborted. The multicenter PACTG 076 Study headed by Dr. Ed Conner nationally and Dr. Pat Flynn for the St. Jude participation randomized HIV-infected women to receive the antiretroviral drug AZT (azidothymidine, Zidovudine) or placebo during the pregnancies. The results reported in the *New England Journal of Medicine 331:1173-80, 1994* showed the reduction of HIV-infected offspring from 28% in the control group to 8 % in the AZT- treated group.

Because of the convincing results of PACTG 076 the administration of AZT to HIV-infected pregnant women became a standard of practice in the U. S. which led to the drastic reduction of Pediatric AIDS as shown in **(FIG. 18-C).**

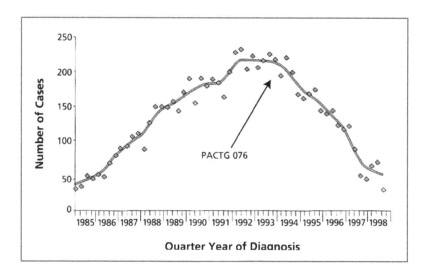

FIG. 18-C: This graph shows the number of perinatally acquired AIDS cases in the United States by year, increasing from 49 cases in 1985 to more than 220 cases in 1994. The arrow points to the time of the PACTG 076 report in 1994. Note the dramatic drop in number of infants with AIDS to less than 50 cases by 1998. (from Vermund, SH. *Top HIV Med 2004: 12 (5): 130-34).*

Soon after the results of the PACTG 076 began to be applied in practice I had another one of those *Deja vu* feelings all over again. We were becoming the victims of our own success in that cases of Pediatric AIDS were diminishing to extent that an adequate number was no longer available for controlled studies – less than 50 cases per year in the whole country and still decreasing rapidly. I was recalling the time described in Chapter 14 when we had eliminated our opportunity for new clinical trials of PCP because of the use of TMP-SMZ prophylaxis.

What to do? I was soon to face in **1996** preparing the renewal of our NIH-PACTG grant, based in great part on clinical trials in Pediatric AIDS. Certainly much more research had to yet be done, but the core of our operation required a substantial number of cases. Already in the NIH Adult ACTG counterpart to PACTG rumblings were being heard about the excessive money being funneled to Pediatrics (meetings were held in Washington and I was there) and that we should not be funded without patients and our funds should be diverted to Adult studies.

In the application for renewal we expanded the definition of Pediatric AIDS based on the American Academy of Pediatrics definition of Pediatrics (from birth to age 21 years). As perinatal AIDS was diminishing HIV infection was increasing in adolescents due to drug abuse and unprotected sex. By expanding Pediatric AIDS to include patients up to age 21 years we could justify continued existence but in doing so would encounter many difficulties in dealing with this age group. Nevertheless, this was where the problems were and our goals had always been to resolve medical problems through research. So, in **1997** our NIH-PACTG Grant was renewed for another four years in the amount of $ 4,505,078.00 with attention to Adolescent AIDS and with Dr. Pat Flynn to serve as Principal Investigator upon my retirement in 1998.

In **1995** I suddenly reached the age of 65 years. A policy had been practiced at St, Jude for Department Chairman to step down at age 65 years and one I supported as a young member and even now at age 65 yrs. Directors at St. Jude had stepped down regularly after about ten years in office. I had never fully appreciated the old professor who continued to toddle into the office until a last breath at age 90. So, I complied more because of the wisdom of the move rather than policy. I had excellent people in our department with organization that would not suffer from my absence as Chairman. However, I was not ready to quit work so I continued as Member and Arthur Ashe Chair for Pediatric AIDS Research until **1998** when I retired.

RETIREMENT – 1998

I hope you children, grandchildren and friends will someday reach a time for retirement. Take good care of yourselves, eat well and stay active until you reach the magic age; after that you can do what you want. It's a time when everyone says nice things about you and you often get some kind of present. I've been told, and I believe it, there has never been a retirement event, party, dinner or other, where anyone ever said anything unpleasant about the honoree, at least anything that was audible. It's the only time in your life this will happen except at your funeral, and you won't know about that. Seriously, I've come to believe that what is said and expressed at these events are from truly genuine feelings and should supersede any prior experiences. I was blessed with two events related to retirement – once when I stepped down as Chairman in **1995** and secondly when I retired "cold turkey" in **1998**.

When I stepped aside (better word than "down"; "up" might be even better) from **Chairman in 1995 Jeanette and I were honored at the National ALSAC Meeting in St. Louis,** with nice comments by Dr. Sam Katz from Duke U. (Scientific Advisory Board), Dr. Arthur Nienhuis (Director St. Jude} and Mr. Richard Shadyac, Sr. (National Executive Director ALSAC). The Board of Governors announced the commission of my portrait for the St. Jude lobby **(FIG. 18-C)**. Danny Thomas' children, Tony, Terre and Marlo, enhanced the honor **(FIG. 18-D)**.

I continued for three more years as an active member, Arthur Ashe Chair for Pediatric AIDS Research and Principle Investigator of the St. Jude PACTG until my RETIREMENT in 1998.

Pat Flynn, MD became Acting Chairman from 1995 to 1997 when **Elaine Toumanen, MD** from Rockefeller University in NY was appointed my successor as Chairman. In 1998 Pat Flynn became the PI for the St. Jude PACTG Grant and in 2002 was appointed as the second recipient of the Arthur Ashe Chair for Pediatric AIDS Research.

In **1998** upon the recommendation of Dr. Neinhuis, I was elected by the Board of Governors to **Emeritus** status of the St. Jude faculty, providing me an indefinite tie to the institution with office and secretarial assistance.

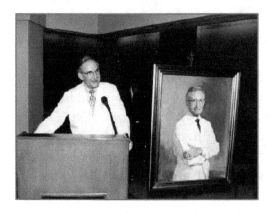

FIG. 18-D: Unveiling of portrait in lobby of St. Jude. Artist Tom Donovan.

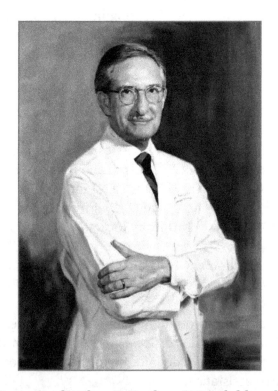

FIG. 18-E: Portrait of Walter T. Hughes, MD in lobby of St. Jude Children's Research Hospital, Artist Tom Donovan.

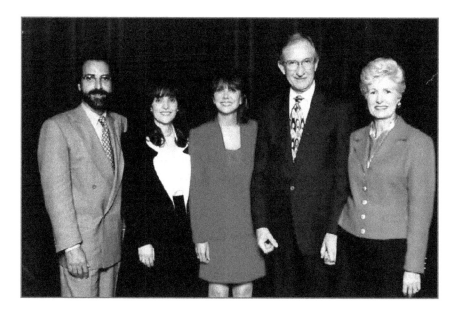

FIG. 18-F: At ALSAC retirement recognition in St. Louis – Tony, Terre and Marlo Thomas, Walter and Jeanette Hughes

RETIREMENT AFTER 1998

I decided to stop "cold turkey" my career in medicine after retirement in 1998. It took another three years to wind down and phase out some ongoing projects, complete book chapters and finish terms on committees, etc. I'll mention a couple of events that I held onto.

On January 19, 2000 I received the **Chancellor's Gold Medal from the University of Chile, Santiago,** the highest recognition award of the famous university founded in 1842. It pleased me because it represented the success of a former St. Jude Infectious Diseases Fellow, **Sergio Vargas, MD** (1991 to 1995). After feasibility visits to Chile in **May, 1993** and with the collaboration of Dr. Vargas in **April, 1994** we submitted to the Director of St. Jude a **"Proposal**

For An International Collaborative Research Program in Infectious Diseases of Children Between St. Jude Children's Research Hospital and the University of Chile-Calvo Mackenna Hospital, Santiago, Chile." St. Jude provided initial funding from **1994 to 1997** for this International Research Center for Infectious Diseases in Chile after which the center has supported itself with progressive growth and prestige to present day (2015). Sergio Vargas is now Professor, Biomedical Institute, U. Chile School of Medicine and internationally renowned for his research on *P. carinii* and importantly, a close personal friend.

From **2000 to 2006** I wrote some novels for my own interest including ***The Yellow Martyrs*** (Writer's Club Press, New York, 2000); ***The Last Leaf*** (Writer's Club Press, New York, 2003); ***Ghosts of Misery Island*** (Publish America, LLD, Baltimore, 2006) and published later ***Suffer the Little Children*** (Publish America, LLD, Baltimore, 2011).

By **2006** I was entering a totally new phase of my life. I was free from job responsibilities and financially secure for retirement and able to do **whatever I wished to do**. Without reservation, the remainder of my life was to be totally dedicated to my dear, sweet wife Jeanette, to savor every moment with her, to have no distraction from our time together. By the Grace of God and the unrelenting support of our children, we were able to spend precious years quietly together at home in Harbor Town on the Mississippi River, watching western sunsets until Jeanette's demise on May 8, 2014.

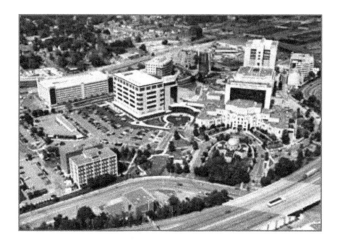

FIG. 18-G: Campus of St. Jude Children's Research Hospital in 2014. All buildings in sight comprise the complex and others are planned or already under construction. The original two-story star-shaped building was just north of the gold dome in lower right; it was demolished and the larger structure built on the site in front of the 1975 building shown in Fig. 13-B.

FUTURE:

At this time I must conclude that the best is yet to come! I look forward to our most beautiful home of all at Chapel Hill Circle, at Elmwood on Dudley Avenue, Memphis, TN 38104. There are no more beautiful scenes in our part of the country than the hills and vales of historic Elmwood Cemetery, founded in 1852. Whether spring, summer, fall or winter Jeanette and I enjoyed excursions there to see the ancient trees, monuments and foliage spread like an artist's canvas before us. This is where we want to reside forever, and so we shall. Our Hughes plots atop the Chapel Hill Circle overlook our favorite terrain and places us within yards of fascinating neighbors such as Dr. John Erskine (honored with St. Jude lectureship}; Miss Ginny Moon, the famous Civil war spy and others I write about in **The Yellow Martyrs**; and the famous Civil War author Shelby Foote and star of Ken Burns' documentary. Here Jeanette waits for me.

When that sweet chariot swings low over the Mississippi co-min' for to carry me home, I'll rise above beloved Harbor Town and St. Jude and make my way to Elmwood to join my precious "Dearie" and to await in time of family to come. (FIG. 18-G-H)

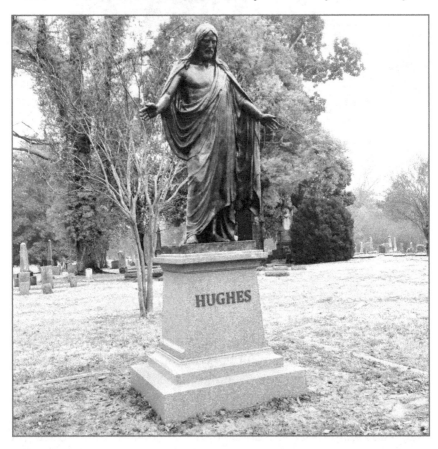

FIG. 18-H: Chapel Hill Circle at Elmwood Cemetery showing Hughes Family plots around monument of *CHRISTUS* created in bronze for Jeanette by Stan Walls, after Thorvaldsen. The first inscription reads "Frances Jeanette Hughes, 'Precious Dearie' December 19, 1930 to May 8, 2014 – Beloved wife, mother and grandmother."

THE END

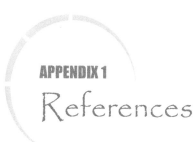

APPENDIX 1

References

REFERENCES TO *Pneumocystis carinii* RESEARCH AT ST. JUDE CHILDREN'S RESEARCH HOSPITAL: 1970 – 2007

Danny Thomas Lecture Series: Walter T. Hughes, M.D. - Nov. 9, 2012

1970s:

1. *Pneumocystis carinii* pneumonia in a hospital for children: epidemiologic aspects.
    Perera DR, Western WA, Johnson HD, Johnson WW, Schultz MG, Akers MA
    JAMA 1970; 214: 1074-78.

2. Recurrent *Pneumocystis carinii* pneumonia following apparent recovery.
    Hughes WT, Johnson WW
    J Pediatr 1971; 79: 755-9.

3. A rapid staining technique for *Pneumocystis carinii*.
    Smith JW, **Hughes WT**
    J Clin Pathol 1972; 25: 269-71.

4. Studies of morphology and immunofluorescence of *Pneumocystis carinii*.
Kim HK, **Hughes WT,** Feldman S.
Proc Soc Exper Biol Med 1972; 141: 304-9.

5. Comparison of methods for identification of *Pneumocystis carinii* in pulmonary aspirates.
Kim HK, **Hughes WT**
Amer J Clin Pathol 1973; 60: 60-462-6.

6. Attempts at prophylaxis for murine *Pneumocystis carinii* pneumonitis.
Hughes WT, Kim HK, Price RA, Miller C
Curr Ther Res Clin Exp 1973; 15: 581-7.

7. Pneumocystis carinii in children with malignancies.
Hughes WT, Price RA, Kim HK, Coburn TP, Grigsby D, Feldman S
J Pediatr 1973; 82: 404.

8. Histopathology of *Pneumocystis carinii* infestation and infection in malignant disease in childhood.
Price RA, **Hughes WT**
Human Pathol 1974; 5: 737-52.

9. Continuous negative chest-wall pressure as therapy for severe respiratory distress in an older child: preliminary observations.
Sanyal SK, MacGaw D, **Hughes WT**
J Pediatr 1974; 85: 230-2.

10. Protein-calorie malnutrition, a host determinant for *Pneumocystis carinii* pneumonitis.
Hughes WT, Price RA, Sisko F, Havron WS, Kafatos AG, Schonland M, Smythe PM.
Amer J Dis Child 1974; 128: 44- 52.

11. Efficacy of trimethoprim-sulfamethoxazole in the prevention and treatment of *Pneumocystis carinii* pneumonitis.
    Hughes WT, McNabb PC, Makres TD, Feldman S
    Antimicrob Agents Chemother 1974; 5: 289-93.

12. Current status of laboratory diagnosis of *Pneumocystis carinii* pneumonitis.
    Hughes WT
    CRC Crit Rev Clin Lab Sci 1975; 6: 145-70.

13. Continuous negative chest-wall pressure as therapy for severe respiratory distress in older children.
    Sanyal SK, Mitchell C, **Hughes WT,** Feldman S, Caces J
    Chest 1975; 68: 143-8.

14. Treatment of *Pneumocystis carinii* pneumonitis with trimethoprim-sulfasmethoxazole.
    Hughes WT, Feldman S, Sanyal SK
    Canad Med Assoc J 1975; 112: (13 spec no.) 37-50.

15. The effect of dimethyl sulfoxide on *Pneumocystis carinii*.
    Smith JW, **Hughes WT**
    Ann NY Acad Sci 1975; 243; 278.

16. Signs, symptoms and pathophysiology of *Pneumocystis carinii* pneumonitis.
    Hughes WT, Sanyal SK, Price A.
    Natl Cancer Inst Monogr 1976; 43: 77-88.

17. Editorial: Treatment of *Pneumocystis carinii* pneumonitis.
    Hughes WT
    N Engl J Med 1976; 295: 726-7.

18. Protozoan infections in haematological disease.
    Hughes WT
    Clin Haematol 1976; 5: 329-45.

19. Infections during continuous complete remission of acute lymphocytic leukemia during and after anticancer therapy.
    Hughes WT
    Int J Radiat Oncol Biol Phys 1976; 1: 305-7.

20. Intensity of immunosuppressive therapy and the incidence of *Pneumocystis carinii* pneumonitis.
    Hughes WT, Feldman S, Aur RJ, Verzosa MS, Hustu HO, Simone JV.
    Cancer 1975; 36: 2004-9.

21. Successful use of continuous negative chest-wall pressure for severe respiratory distress in adults.
    Sanyal SK, Bernal R, **Hughes W**, Feldman S.
    JAMA 1976; 236: 1727.

22. Successful chemoprophylaxis for *Pneumocystis carinii* pneumonitis.
    Hughes WT, Kuhn S, Chaudhary S, Feldman S, Verzosa M, Aur RJ, Pratt C, George S.
    N Engl J Med 1977; 297: 1419-26.

23. *Pneumocystis carinii* pneumonia.
    Hughes WT
    N Engl J Med 1977; 297: 1381-3.

24. Percutaneous transthoracic aspiration of the lung: diagnosing *Pneumocystis carinii* pneumonitis.
    Chaudhary SC, **Hughes WT,** Feldman S, Sanyal SK, Coburn T, Ossi M, Cox F.
    Amer J Dis Child 1977; 131: 902-7.

25. Continuous negative chest-wall pressure therapy for assisting ventilation in older children with progressive respiratory insufficiency.
Sanyal SK, Avery TL, Thapar MK, **Hughes WT**, Harris KS.
Acta Paediatr Scand 1977; 66: 451.

26. Management of severe respiratory insufficiency due to *Pneumocystis carinii* pneumonia in immunosuppressed hosts: the role of continuous negative pressure ventilation.
Sanyal SK, Avery TL, **Hughes WT,** Kumar MA, Harris KS.
Amer Rev Respir Dis 1977; 116: 223-31.

27. Propagation of Pneumocystis carinii in vitro
Pifer LL, **Hughes WT,** Murphy MJ Jr
Pediatr Res 1977; 11: 305-16.

28. Pneumocystis carinii in vitro: study by scanning electron microscopy.
Murphy MJ Jr, Pifer LL, **Hughes WT**
Amer J Pathol 1977; 86: 387-401.

29. Comparison of gastric contents to pulmonary aspirates for the cytologic diagnosis of Pneumocystis carinii pneumonia.
Chan H, Pifer LL, **Hughes WT,** Feldman S, Pearson TA, Woods D.
J Pediatr 1977; 90; 243-4.

30. Pneumocystis carinii pneumonia: a plague of the immunosuppressed.
Hughes WT
Johns Hopkins Med J 1978; 143:184-92.

31. Propagation of *Pneumocystis carinii* in Vero cell culture.
Pifer LL, Woods D, **Hughes WT**
Infect Immun 1978; 20; 66-8.

32. Comparison of pentamidine isethionate and trimethoprim-sulfamethoxazole in the treatment of *Pneumocystis carinii* pneumonia.
     Hughes WT, Feldman S, Chaudhary SC, Ossi MJ, Cox F, Sanyal SK.
     J Pediatr 1978; 92: 285-91.

33. *Pneumocystis carinii* infection: evidence for high prevalence in normal and immunosuppressed children.
     Pifer LL, **Hughes WT,** Stagno S, Woods D
     Pediatr 1978; 61: 35-41.

34. Limited effect of trimethoprim-sulfamethoxazole prophylaxis on *Pneumocystis carinii.*
     Hughes WT
     Antimicrob Agents Chemother 1979; 16: 333-5.

1980s

35. Chemoprophylaxis for *Pneumocystis carinii* pneumonitis: outcome of unstructured delivery.
     Wilber RB, Feldman S, Malone WJ, Ryan M, Aur RJ, **Hughes WT**
     Amer J Dis Child 1980; 134: 643-8.

36. *Pneumocystis carinii* pneumonitis in immunocompetent infants.
     Stagno S, Pifer LL, **Hughes WT,** Brasfield DM, Tiller RE
     Pediatrics 1980; 66; 56-62.

37. Measurement of *Pneumocystis carinii* antigen by enzyme immunoassay.
     Leggiadro RJ, Yolken RH, Simkins JH, **Hughes WT**
     J Infect Dis 1981; 144: 484.

38. Course of pulmonary dysfunction in children surviving *Pneumocystis carinii* pneumonitis.
Sanyal SK, Mariencheck WC, **Hughes WT,** Parvey LS, Tsiatis AA, Mackert PW
Amer Rev Respir Dis 1981; 124: 161-6.

39. Prevalence of *Pneumocystis carinii* pneumonitis in severe combined immunodeficiency.
Leggiadro RJ, Winkelstein JA, **Hughes WT**
J Pediatr 1981; 99: 96-98.

40. Pneumocystis carinii pneumonitis.
Hughes WT
Antibiot Chemother 1981; 30: 257-71.

41. Provocation of infection due to *Pneumocystis carinii by* cyclosporine A.
Hughes WT, Smith BL
J Infect Dis 1982; 145: 767.

42. Trimethoprim-sulfamethoxazole therapy for *Pneumocystis carinii* pneumonia in children.
Hughes WT
Rev Infect Dis 1982; 4: 602-7.

43. Natural mode of acquisition for *de novo* infection with *Pneumocystis carinii.*
Hughes WT
J Infect Dis 1982; 145: 842-8.

44. Provocation of infection due to *Pneumocystis carinii by* cyclosporine A.
Hughes WT, Smith BL
J Infect Dis 1982; 145: 767.

45. <u>Trimethoprim-sulfamethoxazole therapy for *Pneumocystis carinii* pneumonia in children.</u>
    Hughes WT
    Rev Infect Dis 1982; 4: 602-7.

46. <u>Intermittent chemoprophylaxis for *Pneumocystis carinii* pneumonia.</u>
    Hughes WT, Smith BL
    Antimicrob Agents Chemother 1983; 24: 300-1.

47. <u>Rifampicin for *Pneumocystis carinii* pneumonia.</u>
    Hughes WT
    Lancet 1983; 16: 162.

48. <u>A natural source of infection due to *Pneumocystis carinii.*</u>
    Hughes WT, Bartley DL, Smith BL
    J Infect Dis 1983; 147: 595.

49. <u>Efficacy of diaminodiphenylsulfone and other drugs in murine *Pneumocystis carinii* pneumonitis.</u>
    Hughes WT, Smith BL
    Antimicrob Agents Chemother 1984; 26: 436-40.

50. <u>Five-year absence of *Pneumocystis carinii* pneumonitis in a pediatric oncology center.</u>
    Hughes WT
    J Infect Dis 1984; 150: 305-6.

51. <u>Pneumocystis carinii pneumonitis.</u>
    Hughes WT
    Chest 1984; 85: 810-3.

52. <u>Persistence of *Pneumocystis.*</u>
    Hughes WT
    Chest 1985; 88: 4-5.

53. Surfactant phospholipids and lavage phospholipase A2 in experimental *Pneumocystis carinii* pneumonitis.
    Sheehan, PM, Stokes DC, Yeh YY, **Hughes WT**
    Amer Rev Resp Dis 1986; 134: 526-31.

54. Development of murine monoclonal antibodies in *Pneumocystis carinii.*
    Gigliotti F, Stokes DC, Cheatham AB, Davis DS, **Hughes WT.**
    J Infect Dis 1986; 154: 315-22,

55. Lung mechanics, radiography, and 67Ga scintigraphy in experimental *Pneumocystis carinii* pneumonia.
    Stokes DC, **Hughes WT,** Alderson PO, King RE, Garfinkel DJ.
    Br J Exper Pathol 1986; 67: 383-93.

56. Effects of sulfonylurea on *Pneumocystis carinii.*
    Hughes WT, Smith-McCain BL
    J Infect Dis 1986; 153: 944-7.

57. Successful treatment and prevention of murine *Pneumocystis carinii* pneumonia with 4,4'-sulfonylbisformanilide.
    Hughes WT, Smith BL, Jacobus DP
    Antimicrob Agents Chemother 1986; 29: 509-10.

58. Treatment and prophylaxis of *Pneumocystis carinii* pneumonia.
    Hughes WT
    Parasitol Today 1987; 3:332-5.

59. Pneumocystis carinii pneumonitis.
    Hughes WT
    N Engl J Med; 1987: 1021-3.

60. Pneumonia in the immunocompromised host.
    Hughes WT
    Semin Resp Infect 1987; 2:177-83.

61. Successful intermittent chemoprophylaxis for *Pneumocystis carinii* pneumonia.
    Hughes WT, Rivera GK, Schell MJ, Thornton D, Lott L.
    N Engl J Med 1987; 316:1627-32.

62. Experimental *Pneumocystis carinii* pneumonia in the ferret.
    Stokes DC, Gigliotti F, Rehg JE, Snellgrove RL, **Hughes WT**
    Br J Exper Pathol 1987; 68:267-76.

63. Purification and initial characterization of ferret *Pneumocystis carinii* surface antigen.
    Gigliotti F, Ballou LR, **Hughes WT,** Mosley BD
    J Infect Dis 1988; 158: 848-54.

64. Dapsone treatment of *Pneumocystis carinii* pneumonia in the acquired immunodeficiency syndrome.
    Mills J, Leoung G, Medina I, Hopewell PC, **Hughes WT,** Wofsy C.
    Antimicrob Agents Chemother 1988; 32: 1057-60.

65. Presentation of *Pneumocystis carinii* pneumonia as unilateral hyperlucent lung.
    Stokes DC, Shenep JL, Horowitz ME, **Hughes WT**
    Chest 1988; 94: 201-2.

66. Passive immunoprophylaxis with specific monoclonal antibody confers partial protection against *Pneumocystis carinii* pneumonitis in animal models.
    Gigliotti F, **Hughes WT**
    J Clin Invest 1988; 81: 1666-8.

67. Comparison of doses, intervals and drugs in the prevention of *Pneumocystis carinii* pneumonia.
    Hughes WT
    Antimicrob Agents Chemother 1988; 32: 623-5.

68. Nomenclature for *Pneumocystis carinii.*
    Hughes WT, Gigliotti F

69. *Pneumocystis carinii* taxing taxonomy.
    Hughes WT
    Eur J Epidemiol 1989; 5: 265-9.

70. Animal models for *Pneumocystis carinii* pneumonia.
    Hughes WT
    J Protozool 1989; 36: 41-45.

1990s

71. Weekly dapsone for PCP.
    Hughes WT
    Nurse Stand 1990; 5: 16.

72. Prevention of *Pneumocystis carinii* pneumonia in AIDS patients with weekly dapsone.
    Hughes WT, Kennedy W, Dugdale M, Land MA, Stein DS, Weems JJ Jr, Palte S, Landcaster D, Gidan-Kovnar S, Morrison RE
    Lancet 1990; 336: 1066.

73. Prevention of *P. carinii* pneumonia.
    Hughes WT
    Hosp Pract (Off ED) 1990; 25:33-43.

74. Efficacy of a hydroxynaphthoquinone, 566C80, in experimental *Pneumocystis carinii* pneumonia.
    Hughes WT, Gray V, Gutteridge WE, Latter VS, Pudney M
    Antimicrob Agents Chemother 1990; 34: 225-8.

75. Safety and pharmacokinetics of 566C80, a hydroxynaphtho-quinone with anti-*Pneumocystis carinii* activity: a phase 1 study in human immunodeficiency virus (HIV)-infected men.
    Hughes WT, Kennedy W, Shenep JL, Flynn PM, Hetherington SV, Fullen G, Lancaster DJ, Stein DS, Palte S, Rosenbaum D, Liao SHT, Blum R, Rogers M
    J Infect Dis 1991; 163: 843-8.

76. *Pneumocystis carinii*: from Bristol to Bozeman.
    Hughes WT
    J Protozool 1991; 38: 2S.

77. Prevention and treatment of *Pneumocystis carinii* pneumonia.
    Hughes WT
    Ann Rev Med 1991; 42: 287-95.

78. Macrolide-antifol synergism in *Pneumocystis carinii.*
    Hughes W
    J Protoozol 1991; 38: 160S.

89. From the National Institutes of Health. Summary of the Workshop on the future directions in the discovery and development of therapeutic agents for opportunistic infections associated with AIDS.
    Laughon BE, Allaudeen HS, Becker JM, Current WL, Feinberg J, Frenkel JK, Hafner R, **Hughes WT**, Laughlin CA, Meyers JD, et al.
    J Infect Dis 1991; 10: 391-9.

80. *Pneumocystis carinii* pneumonia; new approaches to diagnosis, treatment and prevention.
    Hughes WT
    Pedatr Infect Dis J 1991; 391-9.

81. A preliminary evaluation of 566C80 for the treatment of *Pneumocystis* pneumonia.
    Falloon J, Kovacs J, **Hughes W**, O'Neill D, Polis M, Davey R, Rogers M, LaFon S, Feuerstein I, Lancaster D, Land M, Tuazon C, Dohn M, Greenberg S, Lane HC, Masur H
    N Engl J Med 1991; 325: 1534-1538.

82. Synergistic anti-*Pneumocystis carinii* effects of erythromycin and sulfamethoxazole.
    Hughes WT, Killmar JT
    J Acquir Immune Defic Syndr 1991; 4: 532-7.

83. New drug offers alternative treatment for PCP.
    Hughes WT
    Am Fam Physician 1992; 46: 1275-8.

84. A new drug (566C80) for the treatment of *Pneumocystis carinii* pneumonia.
    Hughes WT
    Ann Intern Med 1992; 116: 953-4

85. Prevention of infections in patients with T-cell defects.
    Hughes WT
    Clin Infect Dis 1993; suppl 2: S368-71.

86. Anti-*Pneumocystis carinii* activity of PS-15, a new biguanide folate antagonist.
    Hughes WT, Jacobus DP, Canfield C, Killmar J
    Antimicrob Agents Chemother 1993; 37: 1417-9.

87. Opportunistic infections in AIDS patients: current management and prevention.
    Hughes WT
    Post Grad Med 1994; 95: 81-2; 85-8, 93.

88. <u>Genetic diversity in human-derived *Pneumocystis carinii* isolates from four geographical locations shown by analysis of mitochondrial rRNA gene sequences.</u>
    Wakefield AE, Fritscher CC, Malin AS, Gwanzura L, **Hughes WT**, Miller RF
    J Clinical Microbiol 1994; 32: 2959-61.

89. <u>Relative potency of 10 drugs with anti-*Pneumocystis carinii* activity in an animal model.</u>
    Hughes WT, Killmar J, Oz HS
    J Infect Dis 1994; 170: 906-11.

90. *Pneumocystis carinii*: <u>what is it and from whence does it come?</u>
    Hughes WT
    J Eukaryot Microbiol 1994; 41: 123S.

91. <u>Prevenion of *Pneumocystis carinii* pneumonia in children with cancer.</u>
    Pui CH, **Hughes WT**, Evans WE, Crist WM
    J Clin Oncol 1994; 12: 1522-3.

92. <u>Sequential changes in vital signs and acid-base and blood-gas profiles in *Pneumocystis carinii* pneumonitis in children with cancer: basis for a scoring system to identify patients who will require ventilator support.</u>
    Sanyal SK, Chebib FS, Gilbert JR, **Hughes WT**
    Amer J Resp Crit Care Med 1994; 149: 1092-8.

93. *Pneumocystis* <u>in infants and children.</u>
    Hughes WT
    N Engl J Med 1995; 333: 320-1.

94. Preventing *Pneumocystis carinii* pneumonia in persons infected with the human immunodeficiency virus.
     Simonds RJ, **Hughes WT,** Feinberg J. Navin TR
     Clin Infect Dis 1995; suppl 1: S44-8.

95. Limited persistence in and subsequent elimination of *Pneumocystis carinii* from the lungs after *P. carinii* pneumonia.
     Vargas SL, **Hughes WT,** Wakefield E, Oz HS
     J Infect Dis 1995; 172: 506-10

96. Adverse events associated with trimethoprim-sulfamethoxazole and atovaquone during the treatment of AIDS- related *Pneumocystis carinii* pneumonia.
     Hughes WT, LaFon SW, Scott JD, Masur H
     J Infect Dis 1995; 171: 1295-301.

97. The role of atovaquone tablets in treating *Pneumocystis carinii* pneumonia.
     Hughes WT
     J Acquir Immune Defic Synd Hum Retrovirol 1995; 8: 247-52.

98. Monodrug efficies of sulfonamides in prophylaxis for *Pneumocystis carinii pneumonia.*
     Hughes WT, Killmar J
     Antimicrob Agents Chemo 1996; 40: 962-5,

99. Search for extrapulmonary *Pneumocystis carinii* in an animal model.
     Oz HS, **Hughes WT**, Vargas SL
     J Parasitol 1996; 82: 357-59.

100. Effect of sex and dexamethasone dose on the experimental host for *Pneumocystis carinii.*
     Oz HS, **Hughes WT**
     Lab Anim Sci 1996; 46: 109-10.

101. Recent advances in the prevention of *Pneumocystis carinii pneumonia.*
   Hughes WT
   Adv Pediatr Infect Dis 1996; 11: 163-86.

102. *Pneumocystis carinii* infection alters GTP-binding proteins in the lung.
   Oz HS, **Hughes WT**
   J Parasitol 1997; 83:679-85.

103. Novel anti-*Pneumocysttis carinii* effects of the immunosuppressant mycophenolate mofetil in contrast to provocative effects of tacrolimus, sirolimus and dexamethasone
   Oz HS, **Hughes WT**
   J Infect Dis 1997; 175: 901-4.

104. Efficacy of lasalocid against murine *Pneumocystis carinii pneumonia.*
   Oz HS, **Hughes W,** Rehg J
   Antimicrobial Agents Chemo 1997; 41: 191-2.

105. Current issues in the epidemiology, transmission, and reactivation of *Pneumocystis carinii.*
   Hughes WT
   Semin Respir Infect 1998; 13: 283-8.

106. Use of dapsone in the prevention and treatment of *Pneumocystis carinii* pneumonia: a review.
   Hughes WT
   Clin Infect Dis 1998; 27:191-204.

107. Effects of aerosolized synthetic surfactant, atovaquone, and the combination of these on murine *Pneumocystis carinii* pneumonia.
> **Hughes WT**, Sillos EM, LaFon S, Rogers M, Wolley JL, Davis C, Studenberg S, Pattishall E, Freeze T, Snyder G, Staton S
> J Infect Dis 1998; 177: 1046-56.

108. A phase 1 safety and pharmacokinetics study of micronized atovaquone in human immunodeficiency virus (HIV)-infected infants and children.
> **Hughes WT**, Dorenbaum A, Yogev R, Beauchamp B, Xu J, McNammara J, Moye J, Purdue L, van Dyke R, Rogers M, Sadler B
> Antimicrob Agents Chemother 1998; 42: 1315.

109. Pharmacokinetics of azithromycin administered with atovaquone in HIV-infected children.
> Ngo LY, Yogev R, Dankner WM, **Hughes WT**, Burchett S, Xu J, Sadler B, Unadkat JD, and ACTG Team.
> Antimicrob Agents Chemother 1999; 43: 1516-1519.

110. Association of *Pneumocystis carinii* and sudden death syndrome.
> Vargas SL, Ponce CA, **Hughes WT**, Wakefield A, Weitz JC, Donoso S, Ulloa AV, Madrid P, Gould S, Latome JJ, Avila R, Benveniste S, Gallo M, Belletti J, Lopez R
> Clin Infect Dis 1999; 29: 1489-93.

111. DNA amplification of nasopharyngeal aspirates in rats: a procedure to detect *Pneumocystis carinii*.
> Oz HS, **Hughes WT**
> Microb Pathog 1999; 27:119-21.

112. Rat model for dual opportunistic prophylaxis: *Cryptosporidium parvum* and *Pneumocystis carinii.*
    Oz HS, **Hughes WT**, Regh JE
    Lab Animal Sci 1999; 49: 331-4.

2000s

113. A rat model for combined *Trypanosoma cruzi* and *Pneumocystis carinii* infection.
    Oz HS, **Hughes WT,** Varilek GW
    Microb Pathog 2000; 29: 187-90.

114. Effect of CD-4 Ligand and other immunomodulators on *Pneumocystis carinii* infection in the rat model.
    Oz HS, **Hughes WT**, Rehg JE, Thomas UK
    Microb Pathog 2000; 29: 187-90

115. Search for *Pneumocystis carinii* DNA in the upper and lower respiratory tracts of humans.
    Oz HS, **Hughes WT**
    Diag Microbiol Infect Dis 2000; 37: 161-4.

116. Transmission of *Pneumocystis carinii* DNA from a patient with *P. carinii* pneumonia to immunocompetent health care workers.
    Vargas SL, Ponce C, Gigliotti F, Ulloa AV, Prieto S, Munoz P, **Hughes W**
    J Clin Microbiol 2000; 38: 1536-8.

117. Provocative effects of the immunosuppressants rapamycin, tacrolimus, and dexamethasone on *Pneumocystis carinii* pneumonitis in contrast to the anti- PCP effects of mycophenolate mofetil.
    Oz HS, **Hughes WT,** Variek G
    Transplantation 2001; 72:1464-5

118. Search for primary infection by *Pneumocystis carinii* in a cohort of normal, healthy infants.
     Vargas SL, **Hughes WT,** Santolaya ME ,Ulloa AV, Ponce CA, Cabrera CE, Cumsillie F, Gigliotti F
     Clinic Infect Dis 2001; 32: 855-61.

119. The effects of atovaquone on etoposide pharmacokinetics in children with acute lymphoblastic leukemia.
     van de Poll MEC, Relling MV, Schuetz EG, Harrison PL, **Hughes WT**, Flynn PM
     Cancer Chemother Pharmacol 2001; 47: 467-72.

120. Pneumocystis carinii vs. Pneumocystis jirovecii: another misnomer (response to Stringer, et al).
     Hughes WT
     Emerg Infect Dis 2003; 9:276-7.

121. Comparison of atovaquone and azithromycin with trimethoprim-sulfamethoxazole for the prevention of serious bacterial infections in children with HIV infection.
     Hughes WT, Dankner WM, Yogev R, Huang S, Paul ME, Flores MA, Kline MW, Wei LJ, PACTG 254 team.
     Clin Infect Dis 2005; 40: 136-45.

122. Pneumocystis carinii vs. Pneumocystis jirovecii (jiroveci) Frenkel.
     Hughes WT
     Clin Infect Dis 2006; 42: 1211-2.

123. Transmission of Pneumocystis species among renal transplant recipients.
     Hughes WT
     Clin Infect Dis 2007; 44: 1150-1.

124. <u>Prophylaxis of Pneumocystis carinii with atovaquone in children with leukemia.</u>
Madden RM, Pui CH, **Hughes WT**, Flynn PM, Leung W
Cancer 2007; 15: 1654-8.

Curriculum Vitae:
Walter T. Hughes, MD

NAME: WALTER T. HUGHES, M.D.

DATE AND PLACE OF BIRTH: May 16, 1930
                                          Cleveland, Tennessee

ACADEMIC DEGREES:

M.D. 1954 University of Tennessee College of Medicine

POSITIONS:

1954-55   Intern, General Hospital, Knoxville, Tennessee
1955-57   Resident, Pediatrics, University of Tennessee
          College of Medicine, LeBonheur Children's Hospital,
          Memphis, Tennessee
1957-59   Staff, Walter Reed Army Medical Unit, Fort Detrick,
          Maryland
1959-61   Private Practice, Pediatrics, Cleveland, Tennessee
1961-62   Instructor in Child Health, University of Louisville
          School of Medicine, Louisville, Kentucky

1962-64   Assistant Professor of Pediatrics, University of Louisville, Louisville, Kentucky

1963-69   Chief of Pediatrics, Louisville General Hospital and Director of Infectious Disease Unit, University of Louisville, Louisville, Kentucky

1964-66   Associate Professor of Pediatrics, University of Louisville, Louisville, Kentucky

1966-69   Professor of Pediatrics, University of Louisville, Louisville, Kentucky

1968-69   Acting Chairman, Department of Pediatrics, University of Louisville, Louisville, Kentucky

1969-77   Chief of Infectious Diseases, St. Jude Children's Research Hospital and Professor of Microbiology and Pediatrics, University of Tennessee, Memphis, Tennessee

1977-81   Eudowood Professor of Pediatric Infectious Diseases, Director of Division of Infectious Diseases, the Johns Hopkins University School of Medicine, Baltimore, Maryland

1981-95   Chairman and Member, Department of Infectious Diseases, St. Jude Children's Research Hospital

1993-98   Arthur Ashe Chair in Pediatric AIDS Research, St. Jude Children's Research Hospital

1981   Professor of Pediatrics (to 2004), and Professor of Preventive Medicine, Division of Biostatistics and Epidemiology (to 1991), University of Tennessee, Memphis, Tennessee.

1981 to   Lecturer in Pediatrics, Johns Hopkins University School of Medicine, Baltimore, Present Maryland

1998 to   Emeritus Member, Department of Infectious Diseases, St. Jude Children's Research

Present   Hospital

SOCIETIES:

Society for Pediatric Research (Emeritus)
Fellow, American Academy of Pediatrics
American Society for Microbiology
Infectious Diseases Society of America
American Pediatric Society
Society of Hospital Epidemiologists of America
Pediatric Infectious Diseases Society (president, 1983-1985)
International AIDS Society
American Medical Association
Immunocompromised Host Society
Society for Protozoologists

AMERICAN LICENSURE:

Maryland, Tennessee, Kentucky

CERTIFICATION:

1960   American Board of Pediatrics

RESEARCH INTEREST:

Infections in the immunosuppressed host

GRANTS (Since 1983):

National Institutes of Health

1. Principal Investigator: National Institute of Allergy and Infectious Diseases AI20673
    April 1983 to April 1986
    Direct costs = $179,038

1 July 1986 - 30 June 1989
Direct costs = $181,533

1 July 1989 - 30 June 1992
Direct costs = $213,258

1 July 1992 - 30 June 1995
Direct costs = $472,685

2. Principal Investigator: (Project 6) Leukemia Project Grant (Joe V. Simone, M.D., P.I. for LPP Grant)
    Project 6 = $86,505
    1984 - 1987

3. Principal Investigator: National Institute of Allergy and Infectious Diseases
    1-U01-AI32908
        1 March 1992 - 28 February 1997
        Direct costs = $3,280,634
    1-U01-AI32908
        1 March 1997 - 28 February 2001
        Direct costs = $4,505,078

American Foundation for AIDS Research

1. Principal Investigator: PAF/AmFAR Grant No. 500115-10-PG
        1 April 1991 - 31 March 1992
        Direct costs = $63,253

William Randolph Hearst Foundation

1. Principal Investigator: Prevention of Pediatrics AIDS
            1 March 1995 - 28 February 1997
            Direct costs = $50,000

AWARDS:

Ettledorf Alumni Award, 1994

Distinguished Physician Award, 1997, Pediatric Infectious Diseases Society

1997 Outstanding Alumnus, University of Tennessee, Memphis

Chancellor's Medal (Medalla Rectoral), University of Chile, 1999

Facultad de Medicina Award, Universidad de Chile (January 2000)

APON Award (October, 2001)

2004 Citation Award: Infectious Diseases Society of America

Gerald P. Bodey MD Award, MD Anderson Cancer Center, University of Texas

PUBLICATIONS:

1. Hughes WT, Ettledorf JN. Oropharyngeal tularemia. J Pediatr 51:363-366, 1957.

2. Hughes WT, Erickson C, Fleishman W, Ettledorf JN. True hermaphroditism. J Pediatr 52:662-666, 1958.

3. Overholt E, Hughes WT, Hornick R. Challenge of Macaca mulatta with 100,000 Pasturella tularensis organisms by the respiratory route. Studies on Pasturella Tularensis. Section II, 1958 Report of United States Army Medical Unit, U.S. Army

Medical Research and Development Command, Walter Reed Army Medical Center, Ft. Dietrick, Maryland.

4. Overholt E, Eiglesbach H, Hornick R, Hughes WT. Living vaccine and tetracycline therapy evaluations in Macaca mulatta aerosol challenged with 60:300:3,000: and 30,000 cells. Ibid.

5. Gochenour W, Overholt E, Gleiser C, Hornick R, Hughes WT, Sills O, Byron W. Modification by viable vaccine in Macaca mulatta monkeys aerosol challenged with 1,300 and 130,000 cells. Ibid.

6. Meadows RW, Hughes WT, Walker LC, Ettledorf JN. Effects of oral 19-Nortestosterone derivative on growth of premature infants. Am J Dis Child 99:206-211, 1960.

7. Steigman AJ, Hughes WT, Delong H. Mumps 1961 and severe nephritis: annotation. Lancet, p 828, 1961.

8. Hughes WT. Tularemia. J Ky Med Assoc 60:667-668, 1962.

9. Hughes WT. Visceral larva migrans: Case report. J Ky Med Assoc 60:270-272, 1962.

10. Hughes WT. Superstitions and home remedies encountered in present-day pediatric practice. J Ky Med Assoc, 1963.

11. Hughes WT. Tularemia in children. J Pediatr 62:495-502, 1963.

12. Hughes WT. A method of collecting micro blood samples for agar gel diffusion analysis. J Pediatr 62:304-305, 1963.

13. Sanyal SK, Hughes WT, Falkner F. Shigellosis in infancy and childhood: Clinical and cerebrospinal fluid findings. J Pediatr 62:784-785, 1963.

14. Hughes WT. Childhood tularemia (original article). Pediatr Digest 5:4-7, 1963.

15. Hughes WT, Faulkner FT. Infant feeding problems. Clin Pediatr 3:65-67, 1964.

16. Hughes WT. Pediatric procedures. Philadelphia: WB Saunders Co, 208 pages, 1964.

17. Hughes WT, Ettledorf JN. Tularemia. In: Gellis S, Kagan B, eds. Current pediatric therapy. Philadelphia: WB Saunders Co, pp 690-691, 1964.

18. Hughes WT, Ettledorf JN. Rickettsial diseases. In: Gellis SS, Kagan BM, eds. Current pediatric therapy. WB Saunders Co, pp 585-588, 1964.

19. Hughes WT. Oculoglandular tularemia: Transmission from rabbit, through dog and tick to man. Pediatrics 36:270-272, 1965.

20. Hughes WT. The physician image. The Centaur 71:2-4, 1965.

21. Hughes WT. Histoplasma capsulatum and atypical mycobacteria. Am J Dis Child 110:89-91, 1965.

22. Hughes WT, Ettledorf JN. Tularemia. In: Gellis SS, Kagan BM, eds. Current pediatric therapy. WB Saunders Co, pp 690-691, 1964.

23. Hughes WT, Fridman Z. Absorption of oral neomycin in infants and children with gastroenteritis. Curr Ther Res 7:240-243, 1965.

24. Hughes WT, Steigman AJ, Delong HF. Some implications of fatal nephritis associated with mumps. Am J Dis Child 111:297-301, 1965.

25. Lewin RA, Hughes WT. Neisseria subflava infections in children. JAMA 195:821-823, 1966.

26. Hughes WT, Kalmer T. Massive talc aspiration: Successful treatment with dexamethasone. Am J Dis Child 111:653-654, 1966.

27. Hughes WT. Acute upper respiratory tract infections in children. Gen Practitioner 102:103-108, 1966.

28. Hughes WT. Generalized aspergillosis with central nervous system involvement. Am J Dis Child 112:262-265, 1966.

29. Sanyal SK, Hughes WT, Falkner FT. Congenital methemoglobinemia: A rare cause of cyanosis in infancy. Indian Pediatr, 1966.

30. Hughes WT. Kinderaztliche untersuchungs und behandlungstechnik. Stuttgart: George Thieme Verlag, 211 pages, 1966.

31. Hughes WT. Tularemia. In: Gellis S, Kagan B, eds. Current pediatric therapy. 2nd ed. Philadelphia: WB Saunders Co, pp 690-691, 1966.

32. Hughes WT, Wan R. Impetigo contagiosa: Etiology, complications and comparison of therapeutic effectiveness of erythromycin and antibiotic ointment. Am J Dis Child 113:449-453, 1967.

33. Hughes WT. Urinary fungi (original article). Urology Digest 6:25-30, 1967.

34. Hughes WT. Management of mumps. In: Conn H, ed. Current therapy. 13th ed. WB Saunders Co, pp 35-37, 1967.

35. Hughes WT. Chromoblastomycosis: Successful treatment with topical amphotericin B. J Pediatr 71:351-356, 1967.

36. Hughes WT. Complication resulting from intramuscular injection. J Pediatr 70:1011-1013, 1967.

37. Hughes WT. Inactivated measles vaccine: Discontinuance of use. J Ky Med Assoc 66:62, 1968.

38. Hughes WT. Evaluation of methacycline in pneumococcic pneumonia of childhood. South Med J 61:173-176, 1968.

39. Kim MY, Hughes WT. Shigellosis: Complications and associated disease in infants and children. J Ky Med Assoc 66:542-548, 1968.

40. Franco S, Hughes WT, Kim MY. Erythromycin in childhood pneumonias. Curr Ther Res 10:345-353, 1968.

41. Hughes WT. Chromoblastomycosis versus sporotrichosis. J Pediatr 73:253-254, 1968.

42. Laraya-Cuasay LR, Wolfe R, Hughes WT. Acute pancreatitis and hypoglycemia. Clin Pediatr 7:525-528, 1968.

43. Hughes WT, Smith J, Kim MY. Suppression of the histoplasmin reaction with measles and smallpox vaccines. Am J Dis Child 116:402-406, 1968.

44. Hughes WT, Ettledorf JN. Tularemia. In: Gellis S, Kagan B, eds. Current pediatric therapy. 3rd ed. Philadelphia: WB Saunders Co, pp 774-775, 1968.

45. Hughes WT. Impetigo-contagiosa in children. GP 39:78-83, 1969.

46. Hall B, Kmetz D, Hughes WT. Reye's syndrome: An association with A - influenza infection. J Ky Med Assoc 67:269-271, 1969.

47. Hughes WT, Collier RN. Streptococcal pharyngitis: Evaluation of erythromycin, erythromycin-sulfa and sulfamethoxazole (possible antagonism between erythromycin and sulfa). Am J Dis Child 118:700-707, 1969.

48. Hughes WT, Franco S, Oh MHK. Systemic blastomycosis in childhood. Clin Pediatr 8:597-601, 1969.

49. Hughes WT. Deep mycoses. In: Kelley VC, ed. Brenneman-Kelley practice of pediatrics. Hagerstown, MD: Hoeber Medical Division, Harper and Row Publishers Inc, pp 1-20, 1970.

50. Hughes WT, Rathauser V. Rocky Mountain spotted fever in children. (Original article). Pediatr Digest pp 29-33, 1970.

51. Hughes WT. Infections and intrauterine growth retardation. Pediatr Clin North Am 17:119-124, 1970.

52. Hughes WT. Rickettsial disease. In: Gellis S, Kagan B, eds. Current pediatric therapy. 4th ed. WB Saunders Co, pp 886-888, 1970.

53. Hughes WT. Leukemia monitoring with fungal bone marrow cultures. JAMA 218:441-443, 1971.

54. Hughes W. Fatal infections in childhood leukemia. Am J Dis Child 122:283-287, 1971.

55. Hughes W, Johnson WW. Recurrent *Pneumocystis carinii* pneumonia following apparent recovery. J Pediatr 79:755-759, 1971.

56. Hughes W. Disseminated mycoses in childhood leukemia. Proceedings International Congress of Pediatrics 6:263-267, 1971.

57. Hughes WT. Mycotic diseases. In: Hughes JG, ed. Synopsis of pediatrics. 3rd ed. CV Mosby Co, pp 813-818, 1971.

58. Smith JW, Hughes W. A rapid staining technique for *Pneumocystis carinii*. J Clin Path 25:269, 1972.

59. Pearson TA, Mitchell CA, Hughes WT. Aeromas hydrophila septicemia. Am J Dis Child 123:579-582, 1972.

60. Metcalf D, Hughes W. Effects of methotrexate on group A beta hemolytic streptococcal infection. Cancer 30:558-593, 1972.

61. Hughes W, Feldman S. Infections in children with leukemia. Hospital Med 8:67-75, 1972.

62. Kim HK, Hughes W, Feldman S. Studies on morphology and immunofluorescence of *Pneumocystis carinii*. Proc Soc Exp Biol Med 141:304-309, 1972.

63. Brunell PA, Gershon AA, Hughes WT, Riley HD, Smith J. Prevention of varicella in high risk children: A collaborative study. Pediatrics 50:718-722, 1972.

64. Hughes WT. Rickettsial disease. In: Gellis S, Kagan B, eds. Current pediatric therapy. 5th ed. WB Saunders Co, pp 632-634, 1972.

65. Hughes WT, Crozier JW. Thermophilic fungi in the myco-flora of man and environmental air. Mycopath Mycol Appl 49:147-152, 1973.

66. Hughes W. Infectious maladies of children with cancer. Paediatrician 1:298-310, 1972-73.

67. Hughes W, Kim HK. Mycoflora in cystic fibrosis: Some ecologic aspects of *Pseudomonas aeruginosa* and *Candida albicans*. Mycopathologica 50:3, 261-269, 1973.

68. Hughes W, Price R, Kim HK, Coburn T, Grigsby D, Feldman S. *Pneumocystis carinii* pneumonitis in children with malignancies. J Pediatr 82:404-415, 1973.

69. Hughes W, Smith DR. Infections during induction of remission of acute lymphocytic leukemia. Cancer 31:1008-1014, 1973.

70. Feldman S, Hughes W, Kim H. Herpes zoster infection in children with cancer. Am J Dis Child 126:178-184, 1973.

71. Sumners JE, Zee P, Hughes W. Relative safety of intravenous alimentation in patients with cancer and neutropenia. J Pediatr 83:288-290, 1973.

72. Hughes WT. Management of *Pneumocystis carinii* pneumonitis. In: Gellis S, Kagan B, eds. Current pediatric therapy. 6th ed. WB Saunders Co, pp 629-631, 1973.

73. Hughes WT, Kim HK, Price RA, Miller C. Attempts at prophylaxis for murine *Pneumocystis carinii* pneumonitis. Curr Ther Res 15:8, 581-587, 1973.

74. Kim H, Hughes W. Comparison of methods for identification of *Pneumocystis carinii* in pulmonary aspirates. Am J Clin Path 60:462-466, 1973.

75. Hughes W. Infection problems in childhood cancer. Seventh National Cancer Conference Proceedings, American Cancer Society. Philadelphia: JB Lippincott Co, pp 601-604, 1973.

76. Hughes WT. Deep mycoses. In: Kelley VC, ed. Brenneman-Kelley practice of pediatrics. Hagerstown, MD: Hoeber Medical Division, Harper and Row Publishers Inc, pp 1-2, 1974.

77. Hughes W, Feldman S, Cox F. Infections in children with cancer. Pediatr Clin North Am 21:583-615, 1974.

78. Cox F, Hughes WT. Disseminated histoplasmosis and childhood leukemia. Cancer 33:1127-1133, 1974.

79. Hughes WT, McNabb PC, Makres TD, Feldman S. Efficacy of trimethoprim and sulfamethoxazole in preventing and treatment of *Pneumocystis carinii* pneumonitis. Antimicrob Agents Chemother 5:289-293, 1974.

80. Sanyal SK, McGaw D, Hughes WT, Harris S, Rogers A. Continuous negative chest-wall pressure as therapy for severe respiratory distress in an older child. J Pediatr 85:230-236, 1974.

81. Hughes WT, Feldman S, Herman HW. Safety of megadose haloprogin. Arch Dermatol 110:926-928, 1974.

82. Cox F, Hughes WT. Fecal excretion of cytomegalovirus in disseminated cytomegalic inclusion disease. J Infect Dis 129:732-736, 1974.

83. Price RA, Hughes W. Histopathology of *Pneumocystis carinii* infestation and infection in malignant disease of childhood. Human Pathol 5:737-752, 1974.

84. Sanyal SK, McGaw D, Hughes WT, Harris KS. The negative approach. Emergency Medicine 6:241, 1974.

85. Hughes WT, Price RA, Sisko F, Havron S, Kafatos AG, Schonland M, Smythe PM. Protein-calorie malnutrition: a host determinant for *Pneumocystis carinii* infection. Am J Dis Child 128:44-52, 1974.

86. Hughes WT. Mycotic diseases. In, Hughes JG, ed. Synopsis of pediatrics. 4th ed. CV Mosby Co, pp 793-797, 1975.

87. Smith JW, Hughes WT. The effect of dimethyl sulfoxide on *Pneumocystis carinii*. Ann NY Acad Sci 243-278, 1975.

88. Sanyal SK, Mitchell C, Hughes WT, Feldman S, Caces J. Continuous negative chest-wall pressure as therapy for severe respiratory distress in older children. Chest 68:143-148, 1975.

89. Feldman S, Hughes WT, Daniel CB. Varicella in children with cancer: Seventy-seven cases. Pediatrics 56:388-397, 1975.

90. Feldman S, Hughes WT, Darlington RW, Kim HW. Evaluation of topical polyinosinic acid-polycytidylic acid in treatment of localized herpes zoster in children with cancer: A randomized double-blind controlled study. Antimicrob Agents Chemother 8:289-294, 1975.

91. Cox F, Hughes WT. The value of isolation procedures for cytomegalovirus infections in children with leukemia. Cancer 36:1158-1161, 1975.

92. Hughes WT. Current status of laboratory diagnosis of *Pneumocystis carinii* pneumonitis. Crit Rev Clin Lab Sci 6:145-170, 1975.

93. Hughes WT. *Pneumocystis carinii* pneumonitis (editorial). Lancet 2:1023-1024, 1975.

94. Hughes WT, Feldman S, Aur RJA, Verzosa MS, Hustu HO, Simone J. Intensity of immunosuppressive therapy and the incidence of Pneumocystis carinii pneumonitis. Cancer 36:2004-2009, 1975.

95. Hughes WT. Infections in the compromised host. In: Shirkey HC, ed. Pediatric therapy. 5th ed. St. Louis: CV Mosby Co, pp 405-410, 1975.

96. Cox F, Hughes WT. Contagious and other aspects of nocardiosis in the compromised host. Pediatrics 55:135-138, 1975.

97. Cox F, Hughes WT. Cytomegaloviremia in children with acute lymphocytic leukemia. J Pediatr 87:190-194, 1975.

98. Hughes WT, Feldman S, Sanyal SK. Treatment of *Pneumocystis carinii* pneumonitis with trimethoprim-sulfamethoxazole. Can Med Assoc J (Suppl) 112:47-50, 1975.

99. Hughes WT. Infection in children with malignant disease. In: Bloom HJG, Lemerle H, Neidhardt MK, Voute PA, eds. Cancer in children. Berlin: Springer-Verlag, pp 62-71, 1975.

100. Cox F, Meyer C, Hughes WT. Cytomegalovirus in tears from patients with normal eyes and with acute cytomegalovirus chorioretinitis. Am J Dis Child 80:817-824, 1975.

101. Hughes WT. Management of *Pneumocystis carinii* pneumonitis. In: Gellis S, Kagan B, eds. Current pediatric therapy. 7th ed. Philadelphia: WB Saunders Co, pp 589-591, 1976.

102. Hughes WT. Infections in the compromised host. In: Stollerman GH, ed. Advances in internal medicine. Vol 22. Chicago: Yearbook Medical Pub, pp 73-96, 1976.

103. Hughes WT, Sanyal SK, Price RA. Signs, symptoms and pathophysiology of *Pneumocystis carinii* pneumonitis. In: Symposium on *Pneumocystis carinii* infection. National Cancer Institute Monograph, National Institutes of Health, 1976.

104. Hughes WT. Infections in the compromised host. In: Kelley VC, ed. Brennemann-Kelley practice of pediatrics. Chapter 1G, Vol 2. Hagerstown, MD: Hoeber Medical Division of Harper and Row Publishers, Inc, p 1, 1976.

105. Gunasekaran M, Hughes WT, Maguire WJ. Cyclic 3'5' nucleotide phosphodiesterase of *Candida albicans*. Microbios Letters 3:47-53, 1976.

106. Hughes W. Infections during continuous complete remission of acute lymphocytic leukemia: during and after anticancer therapy. Int J Radiol Oncol Phys 1:305-307, 1976.

107. Hughes WT. Early side effects in treatment of childhood cancer. Pediatr Clin North Am 23:225-232, 1976.

108. Patterson TA, Hughes WT, Billmeier GJ, Pearson T. Ampicillin-resistant *Hemophilus influenzae* meningitis. J Tenn Med Assoc pp 99-101, 1976.

109. Hughes WT. Protozoan infection haematological diseases. Clin Haematol 5:329-345, 1976.

110. Gardner SE, Hughes WT, Pearson T. Corynebacterium equi pneumonitis. Chest 70:92-94, 1976.

111. Sanyal SK, Bernal R, Hughes W, Feldman S. Successful use of continuous negative chest-wall pressure for severe respiratory distress in adults. JAMA 236:1727, 1976.

112. Hughes WT. Treatment of *Pneumocystis carinii* pneumonia (editorial). New Engl J Med 295:726-727, 1976.

113. Hughes WT. Mosaic law and infection control. Assoc Pract Infect Control 5:25-27, 1977.

114. Chan H, Pifer L, Hughes WT, Feldman S, Pearson T, Woods D. Comparison of gastric contents to pulmonary aspirates for the cytological diagnosis of *Pneumocystis carinii* pneumonia. J Pediatr 90:243-244, 1977.

115. Pifer L, Hughes WT, Murphy M. Propagation of *Pneumocystis carinii* in vitro. Pediatr Res 11:305-316, 1977.

116. Murphy MJ, Pifer LL, Hughes WT. *Pneumocystis carinii* in vitro: A study by scanning electron microscopy. Am J Pathol 86:387-402, 1977.

117. Sanyal SK, Avery TL, Thapar MK, Hughes WT, Harris KS. Continuous negative chest-wall pressure therapy for assisting ventilation in older children with progressive respiratory insufficiency. Acta Paediatr Scand 66:451-456, 1977.

118. Hughes WT. *Pneumocystis carinii* pneumonia. In: Kendig EL, Chernik V, eds. Disorders of the respiratory tract in children. 3rd ed. Philadelphia: WB Saunders Co, pp 403-411, 1977.

119. Sanyal S, Avery TL, Hughes WT, Kumar M, Harris KS. Management of severe respiratory insufficiency due to *Pneumocystis carinii* pneumonitis in immunosuppressed hosts. Am Rev Respir Dis 16:223-231, 1977.

120. Gunasekaran M, Hughes WT. A simple medium for isolation and identification of *Candida albicans* directly from clinical specimens. Mycopathologica 61:3, 151-157, 1977.

121. Chaudhary S, Hughes WT, Feldman S, Sanyal SK, Coburn T, Ossi M, Cox F. Percutaneous transthoracic needle aspiration of the lung: diagnosing *Pneumocystis carinii* pneumonitis. Am J Dis Child 131:902-907, 1977.

122. Hughes WT. Infection in the immunosuppressed host. In: Rudolph AM, ed. Pediatrics. 16th ed. New York: Appleton-Century Crofts, pp 412-414, 1977.

123. Hughes WT, Kuhn S, Chaudhary S, Feldman S, Verzosa M, Aur RJA, Pratt C, George SL. Successful chemoprophylaxis for *Pneumocystis carinii* pneumonitis. N Engl J Med 297:1419-1426, 1977.

124. Hughes WT. Current concepts: *Pneumocystis carinii* pneumonia. N Engl J Med 297:1381-1383, 1977.

125. Hughes WT. *Pneumocystis carinii* pneumonitis. In: Kelley VC, ed. Brenneman-Kelley practice of pediatrics. Chapter 52B, Vol II. Hagerstown, MD: Hoeber Medical Division of Harper and Row Publishers Inc, pp 1-8, 1977.

126. Hughes WT. Management of *Pneumocystis carinii* pneumonitis. In: Gellis S, Kagan B, eds. Current pediatric therapy. 8th ed. WB Saunders Co, pp 608-610, 1978.

127. Hughes WT. Histoplasmosis. In: Gellis S, Kagan B, eds. Current pediatric therapy. 8th ed. Philadelphia: WB Saunders Co, pp 644-645, 1978.

128. Pifer L, Hughes WT, Stagno S, Woods D. *Pneumocystis carinii* infection: evidence for high prevalence in normal and immunosuppressed children. Pediatrics 61:35-41, 1978.

129. Pifer L, Elliott S, Woodward T, Woods D, Hughes WT. An improved method for detection of *Hemophilus influenzae* b antigen in cerebrospinal fluid. J Pediatr 92:227-229, 1978.

130. Gunasekaran M, Hughes WT. A simple liquid medium for chlamydospore formation in *Candida albicans*. Mycopathologica et Mycologica Appl. 64:143-146, 1978.

131. Pifer LL, Woods D, Hughes WT. Propagation of *Pneumocystis carinii* in Vero cell culture. Infect Immunol 20:66-68, 1978.

132. Hughes WT. Pneumocystis pneumonitis: A plague of the immunosuppressed. Johns Hopkins Med J 143:184-192, 1978.

133. Hughes WT, Feldman S, Chaudhary S, Ossi MJ, Cox F, Sanyal SK. Comparison of pentamidine isethionate and trimethoprim-sulfamethoxazole in the treatment of *Pneumocystis carinii* pneumonia. J Pediatr 92:285-291, 1978.

134. Hughes WT, Kuhn S, Chaudhary S, Feldman S, Verzosa M, Aur R, Pratt CB. Prevention of *Pneumocystis carinii* pneumonitis with trimethoprim- sulfamethoxazole prophylaxis. Current chemotherapy. Vol 1. Proceedings of the 10th International Congress of Chemotherapy. Am Soc Microbiol, Washington, DC, pp 250-251, 1978.

135. Hughes WT. Life-threatening infections in the compromised host. Current chemotherapy. Vol 1. Proceedings of the 10th International Congress of Chemotherapy. Am Soc Microbiol, Washington, DC, pp 37-42, 1978.

136. Cox F, Hughes WT. Gallium-67 scanning for the diagnosis of infection in children. Am J Dis Child 133:1171-1173, 1979.

137. Hughes WT. Limited effect of trimethoprim-sulfamethoxazole prophylaxis on *Pneumocystis carinii*. Antimicrob Agents Chemother 16:333-335, 1979.

138. Chipps BE, Saulsbury FT, Hsu SH, Hughes WT, Winkelstein JA. Non-candidal infections in children with chronic mucocutaneous candidiasis. Johns Hopkins Med J 144:175-179, 1979.

139. Hughes WT. Advances in supportive care: Infection. In: Care of the child with cancer. Philadelphia: George F Stickley Co, pp 101-105, 1979.

140. Hughes WT. *Pneumocystis carinii*. In: Mandell GL, Douglas RG, Bennett JE, eds. Principals and practice of infectious diseases. Chapter 231. John Wiley and Sons, pp 2137-2142, 1979.

141. Hughes WT. *Pneumocystis carinii* pneumonia. In: Schultz MG, ed. Current concepts in parasitology. Boston: Mass Medical Society, pp 32-40, 1979.

142. Hughes WT, Buescher S. Pediatric Procedures. 2nd ed. Philadelphia: WB Saunders Co, pp 367, 1980.

143. Hughes WT. *Pneumocystis carinii* pneumonia. In: The clinical use of sulfamethoxazole/trimethoprim. Amsterdam: Excerpta Medica, pp 115-127, 1980.

144. Bender JW, Hughes WT. Fatal *Staphylococcus epidermidis* sepsis following bone marrow transplantation. Johns Hopkins Med J 146:13-15, 1980.

145. Hughes WT. Sequelae of infectious diseases. In: Faulkner F, ed. Prevention in childhood of specific adult health problems. Geneva: World Health Organization, pp 95-106, 1980.

146. Gunasekaran M, Hughes WT. Gas-liquid chromatography: A rapid method for identification of different *Candida* species. Mycologica 72:505-511, 1980.

147. Hughes WT. *Pneumocystis carinii* pneumonitis. In: Gellis S, Kagan B, eds. Current pediatric therapy. 9th ed. Philadelphia: WB Saunders Co, pp 572-574, 1980.

148. Hughes WT. Infection in the compromised host. In: Shirkey HC, ed. Pediatric therapy. 6th ed. St. Louis: CV Mosby Co, pp 382-387, 1980.

149. Hughes WT. Infections in the compromised host. In: Kelley VC, ed. Practice of pediatrics. Chapter 1G. Hagerstown, MD: Harper & Row Publishers Inc, pp 1-7, 1980.

150. Wilber RB, Feldman S, Malone WJ, Ryan M, Aur RJA, Hughes WT. Outcome of unstructured delivery of chemoprophylaxis for *P. carinii* pneumonitis. Am J Dis Child 134:643-648, 1980.

151. Yolken RH, Hughes WT, Stopa PJ. Rapid diagnosis of infections caused by b-lactamase-producing bacteria by means of an enzyme radioisotopic assay. J Pediatr 97:715-720, 1980.

152. Stagno S, Pifer LL, Hughes WT, Brasfield DM, Tiller RE. *Pneumocystis carinii* pneumonitis in young immunocompetent infants. Pediatrics 66:56-62, 1980.

153. Hughes WT, Fuchs F. Infections affecting the fetus. In: Falkner F, ed. Prevention in Childhood of Health Problems in Adult Life. Geneva: World Health Organization, 1980.

154. Hughes WT. *Pneumocystis carinii* pneumonia. In: Kelley VC, ed. Brenneman-Kelly practice of pediatrics. Chapter 52-B. Hagerstown, MD: Hoeber Medical Division of Harper and Row Publishers Inc, pp 1-8, 1980.

155. Hughes WT, Townsend TR. Nosocomial infections in immuno-suppressed children. Am J Med 70:412-416, 1981.

156. Hughes WT. *Pneumocystis carinii* pneumonia. In: Allen J, ed. Infections in the compromised host. 2nd ed. Williams and Wilkins Co, pp 91-106, 1981.

157. Hughes WT. *Pneumocystis carinii* pneumonia. In: Schonfeld H, ed. Antibiotics and chemotherapy: Antiparasitic chemothera-py. Vol 30. S Karger, pp 256-271, 1981.

158. Leggiadro RJ, Winkelstein JA, Hughes WT. Prevalence of *Pneumocystis carinii* pneumonitis in severe combined immu-nodeficiency. J Pediatr 88:96-98, 1981.

159. Sanyal SK, Mariencheck WC, Hughes WT, Parvey LS, Tsiatis AA, Mackert PW. Course of pulmonary dysfunction in children surviving *Pneumocystis carinii* pneumonitis: A prospective study. Am Rev Respir Dis 124:161-166, 1981.

160. Corrall CJ, Peeple JM, Moxon ER, Hughes WT. C-reactive protein in spinal fluid of children with meningitis. J Pediatr 99:365-369, 1981.

161. Leggiadro RJ, Yolken RH, Simkins JH, Hughes WT. Measurement of *Pneumocystis carinii* antigen by enzyme immunoassay. J Infect Dis 144:484, 1981.

162. Hughes WT, Townsend TR. Nosocomial infections in immunocompromised children. In: Dixon RE, ed. Nosocomial infections. Yorke Medical Books, pp 38-42, 1981.

163. Hughes WT. Immunology of *Pneumocystis carinii*. In: Nahmias AJ, O.Reilly RJ, Good RA ed-in-chief, eds. Immunology of human infection. Part II. New York: Plenum Publishing Co, pp 373-383, 1982.

164. Hughes WT. *Pneumocystis carinii*. In: Barron S, ed. Medical microbiology. Addison-Wesley Publishing Co, pp 785-787, 1982.

165. Hughes WT. Systemic candidiasis: A study of 109 fatal cases. Pediatr Infect Dis 1:11-18, 1982.

166. Hughes WT. Natural mode of acquisition for de novo infection with *Pneumocystis carinii*. J Infect Dis 145:842-848, 1982.

167. Hughes WT, Smith B. Provocation of infection due to *Pneumocystis carinii* by cyclosporin A. J Infect Dis 145:767, 1982.

168. Hughes WT. Drugs for systemic mycoses. Pediatr Infect Dis 1:177-179, 1982.

169. Hughes WT. Trimethoprim-sulfamethoxazole therapy for *Pneumocystis carinii* in children. Rev Infect Dis 4:602-609, 1982.

170. Corrall CJ, Merz WG, Rekedal K, Hughes WT. *Aspergillus* osteomyemyelitis in an immunocompetent adolescent: A case report and review of the literature. Pediatrics 70:455-461, 1982.

171. Hughes WT. Pneumocystis pneumonia. In: Rudolph AM, ed. Pediatrics. 17th ed. New York: Appleton-Century Crofts, pp 707-708, 1982.

172. Hughes WT, Koblin BA, Rosenstein BJ. Lysozyme activity in cystic fibrosis. Pediatr Res 16:874-876, 1982.

173. Bartley DL, Hughes WT, Parvey LS, Parham D. Computed tomography of hepatic and splenic fungal abscesses in leukemic children. Pediatr Infect Dis 1:317-321, 1982.

174. Hughes WT. *Pneumocystis carinii* pneumonia. In: Wedgewood RJ, Davis SD, Ray CG, Kelley VC, eds. Infections in children. Philadelphia: Harper and Row Pub, pp 1400-1408, 1982.

175. Hughes WT. Infections in the compromised host. In: Wedgewood RJ, Davis SD, Ray CG, Kelley VC, eds. Infections in children. Philadelphia: Harper and Row Pub, pp 152-158, 1982.

176. Hughes WT. Infection in the immunosuppressed host. In: Rudolph AM, ed. Pediatrics. 17th ed. New York: Appleton-Century Crofts, pp 487-489, 1982.

177. Hughes WT. Les sequelles des maladies infectieuses de l'enfance. In: Falkner F. Prévention chez l'enfant des problémes de santé du futur adulte. Genéve: Organisation Mondiale de la Sante, pp 109-122, 1982.

178. Hughes WT, Fuchs F. Infections touchant le foetus. In: Falkner R. Prevention chez l'enfant des problémes de santé du futur adulte. Genéve: Organisation Mondiale de la Santa, pp 99-107, 1982.

179. Hughes WT. Trimethoprim-sulfamethoxazole. Pediatr Clin North Am 30:27-30, 1983.

180. Hughes WT, Tufenkeji H, Bartley D. The immune compromised host. Pediatr Clin North Am 30:103-120, 1983.

181. Hughes WT, Bartley DL, Smith BM. A natural source for *Pneumocystis carinii* infection. J Infect Dis 147:595, 1983.

182. Hughes WT, Bartley DL, Patterson G, Tufenkeji H. Ketoconazole and candidiasis: A controlled study. J Infect Dis 147:1060-1063, 1983.

183. Hughes WT. *Pneumocystis carinii*. In: Weatherall DJ, Ledingham JGG, Warrell DA, eds. Oxford textbook of medicine. Oxford: Oxford University Press, pp 5.399-5.400, 1983.

184. Ruskin J, Hughes WT. *Pneumocystis carinii* pneumonia. In: Remington JS, Klein JO, eds. Infectious diseases of the fetus and newborn infant. 2nd ed. Philadelphia: WB Saunders Co, pp 507-543, 1983.

185. Hughes WT. *Pneumocystis carinii* pneumonitis. In: Kendig EL, Chernick R, eds. Disorders of the respiratory tract in children. 4th ed, Chapter 20. WB Saunders Co, pp 314-322, 1983.

186. Hughes WT. Trimethoprim-sulfamethoxazole: 10 questions physicians often ask. Consultant 23:73-82, 1983.

187. Hughes WT. Tuberculosis today. Pediatr Infect Dis 2(5):37-40, 1983.

188. Hughes WT. Fungi: friends and foes. Pediatr Infect Dis 2(5):18-22, 1983.

189. Hughes WT. Neutropenia and fever. Pediatr Infect Dis 2(5):14-17, 1983.

190. Hughes WT, Smith BL. Intermittent chemoprophylaxis for *Pneumocystis carinii* pneumonia. Antimicrob Agents Chemother 24:300-301, 1983.

191. Hughes WT, Buescher ES. Procedimentos técnicos em pediatria. 2nd ed. Rio de Janeiro, Brazil: Interamericana Ltda, pp 1-346, 1983.

192. Hughes WT. Rifampicin for *Pneumocystis carinii* pneumonia (Letter). Lancet 2:162, 1983.

193. Hughes WT. Anti-infective therapy in the immunosuppressed patient. In: MacLeod SM, Okey AB, Spielberg SP, eds. Developmental pharmacology (Progress in Clinical and Biological Research). Vol 1351. New York: Alan R Liss Inc, pp 329-339, 1983.

194. Gunasekaran M, Hughes WT, Wilber RB. Rapid diagnosis of systemic candidiasis in children with cancer by pyrolysis gas liquid chromatography. Mycopathologia 84:17-19, 1983.

195. Hughes WT, Patterson G. Post-sepsis prophylaxis in cancer patients. Cancer 53:137-141, 1984.

196. Hughes WT. Assessing response to therapy for mucosal candidiasis. (Correspondence) J Infect Dis 149:284-285, 1984.

197. Hughes WT. *Pneumocystis carinii* pneumonitis. In: Gellis S, Kagan B, eds. Current pediatric therapy. 10th ed. WB Saunders Co.

198. Hughes WT. *Pneumocystis carinii* pneumonitis. In: Gellis S, Kagan B, eds. Current pediatric therapy. 11th ed. WB Saunders Co, pp 561-563, 1984.

199. Hughes WT. *Pneumocystis carinii* - a model for nutrition-immunity interaction. In: Ogra PL, ed. Neonatal infections: nutritional and immunologic interactions. New York: Grune and Stratton Inc, pp 247-263, 1984.

200. Hughes WT. *Pneumocystis carinii* pneumonitis. Chest 85:810-813, 1984.

201. Hughes WT. Folate antagonists as antiprotozoan agents: Clinical studies. In: Sirotnak FM, Burchall JJ, Ensminger WB, Montgomery JA, eds. Folate antagonists as therapeutic agents. Academic Press, pp 251-269, 1984.

202. Hughes WT. Pneumocystosis. In: Strickland GT, ed. Tropical medicine. 6th ed. Philadelphia: WB Saunders Co, pp 605-608, 1984.

203. Hughes WT. Five-year *Pneumocystis* pneumonitis-free survival in an oncology center. J Infect Dis 150:305-306, 1984.

204. Hughes WT. The origin of *Pneumocystis carinii* (correspondence). J Infect Dis 149:287-289, 1984.

205. Hughes WT. Hematogenous histoplasmosis in the immunocompromised child. J Pediatr 105:569-575, 1984.

206. Hughes WT, Smith BL. Efficacy of diaminodiphenylsulfone and other drugs in murine *Pneumocystis carinii* pneumonitis. Antimicrob Agents Chemother 26:436-440, 1984.

207. Hughes WT. Infections in children with cancer: Part I - most common causes and how to treat them. Primary Care and Cancer. 4:66-72, 1984.

208. Hughes WT. *Pneumocystis carinii*: Biology and mode of transmission. In: Gottlieb MS, Groopman JE, eds. Acquired immune deficiency syndrome. New York: Alan R Liss Inc, pp 345-354, 1984.

209. Hughes WT. Sections on enteroviral infections, mycotic diseases, chlamydia infection and *Pneumocystis carinii* pneumonia. In: Hughes JG, Griffith JF, eds. Synopsis of pediatrics. 6th ed. CV Mosby Co, pp 763-767, 753-760, 1984.

210. Hughes WT. Preventing infections in children: Guidelines for physicians and patients. Primary Care and Cancer 4:58-60, 1984.

211. Enggarro IL, Hughes WT, Kalwinsky DK, Pearson TA, Parham D, Stass SA. Disseminated *Pseudoallescheria boydii* in a patient with acute lymphoblastic leukemia. Arch Pathol Lab Med 108:619-622, 1984.

212. Hughes WT. *Pneumocystis carinii*. In: Mandell GL, Douglas RG, Bennett JE, eds. Principles and practice of infectious diseases. 2nd ed. New York: John Wiley & Sons Inc, pp 1549-1552, 1985.

213. Hughes WT. Infections in the compromised host. In: Kelley VC, ed. Practice of pediatrics. Vol 3, Chapter 13. Harper & Row Pub Inc, pp 1-10, 1985.

214. Hughes WT. *Pneumocystis carinii pneumonia*. In: Kelley VC, ed. Practice of pediatrics. Chapter 57. Harper & Row Pub Inc, pp 1-9, 1985.

215. Hughes WT. Drugs for systemic mycoses. In: Nelson JD, McCracken GH, eds. Clinical reviews in pediatric infectious diseases. St. Louis: CV Mosby Co, pp 59-62, 1985.

216. Hughes WT. Fundamentals of immunization. In: Falkner F, ed. Prevention of infant mortality and morbidity. Basel: S Karger Pub, pp 93-102, 1985.

217. Hughes WT, Feldman S, Gigliotti F, Shenep J, Sixbey J. Prevention of infectious complications in acute lymphoblastic leukemia. Semin Oncol 12(2):180-191, 1985.

218. Feldman S, Doolittle M, Lott L, Roberson P, Hughes WT. Similar hematological changes in children receiving trimethoprim-sulfamethoxazole or amoxicillin for otitis media. J Pediatr 106:995-1000, 1985.

219. Hughes WT, Patterson GG, Thorton D, Williams BJ, Lott L, Dodge R. Detection of fever with infrared thermometry: a feasibility study. J Infect Dis 152:301-306, 1985.

220. Shenep JL, Stokes DC, Hughes WT. Lack of antibacterial activity after intravenous hydrogen peroxide infusion in experimental *Escherichia coli* sepsis. Infect Immun 48(3):607-610, 1985.

221. Hughes WT. Persistence of pneumocystis. Chest 88:4-5, 1985.

222. Hughes WT. Serodiagnosis of *Pneumocystis carinii* (Letter). Chest 87:700, 1985.

223. Hughes WT. *Pneumocystis carinii*. In: Barron S, ed. Medical microbiology. 2nd ed. Menlo Park: Addison-Wesley, pp 1057-1060, 1985.

224. Hughes WT. Nutrition and infection. In: Farber GB, ed. Pediatric nutrition handbook. 2nd ed. Elk Grove, IL: Committee on nutrition, Amer Acad Peds, pp 267-272, 1985.

225. Haponik EF, Stokes D, Rosenstein BJ, Hughes WT. ABH secretor status in cystic fibrosis - a negative report. Eur J Respir Dis 67:381-384, 1985.

226. Hughes WT. *Pneumocystis carinii* pneumonia. In: Gellis S, Kagan B, eds. Current pediatric therapy. 12th ed. pp 567-569, 1986.

227. Hughes WT. Tularemia. In: Gellis S, Kagan B, eds. Current pediatric therapy. 12th ed. WB Saunders Co, pp 550-551, 1986.

228. Hughes WT. Candidiasis. In: Nelson JD, ed. Current therapy in pediatric infectious diseases. Philadelphia: BC Decker Inc Pub, pp 133-134, 1986.

229. Hughes WT. Cryptococcosis. In: Nelson JD, ed. Current therapy in pediatric infectious diseases. Philadelphia: BC Decker Inc Pub, pp 138-139, 1986.

230. Hughes WT. Sulfonamides and trimethoprim. In: Peterson PK, Verhoef J, eds. The antimicrobial agents annual I. Amsterdam: Elsevier Science Pub, pp 197-204, 1986.

231. Hughes WT, Smith BL, Jacobus DP. Successful treatment and prevention of murine *Pneumocystis carinii* pneumonitis with 4,4'sulfonylbisformanilide. Antimicrob Agents Chemother 29:509-510, 1986.

232. Aronoff SC, Hughes WT, Kohl S, Speck WT, Wald ER, eds. Advances in pediatric infectious diseases. Vol I. Yearbook Pub, 1986.

233. Hughes WT. Phycomycoses. In: Nelson JD, ed. Current therapy in pediatric infectious diseases. Philadelphia: BC Decker Inc Pub, pp 143-144, 1986.

234. Hughes WT. Infections in children with malignant disease. In: Voute PA, Barrett A, Bloom G, Lemerle J, Neidhardt MK, eds. Cancer in children, clinical management. 2nd ed. Berlin: Springer-Verlag, pp 60-69, 1986.

235. Stokes DC, Hughes WT, Alderson PO, King RE, Garfinkel DJ. Lung mechanics, radiography and ^{67}Ga scintigraphy in experimental *Pneumocystis carinii* pneumonia. Br J Exp Pathol 67:383-393, 1986.

236. Hughes WT, McCain B. Effects of sulfonylurea compounds on *Pneumocystis carinii*. J Infect Dis 153:944-947, 1986.

237. Sheehan PM, Stokes DC, Yeh Y-Y, Hughes WT. Surfactant phospholipids and lavage phospholipase A_2 in experimental *Pneumocystis carinii* pneumonia. Am Rev Respir Dis 134:526-531, 1986.

238. Hughes WT. Recent advances in serodiagnosis of *Pneumocystis carinii* (Response Commun to editor). Chest 89:765, 1986.

239. Hughes WT. *Pneumocystis carinii* pneumonitis. In: Levin MJ, ed. The immunocompromised host. World Health Comm NY 3(5):1-11, 1986.

240. Gigliotti F, Stokes DC, Cheatham AB, Davis DS, Hughes WT. Development of murine monoclonal antibodies to *Pneumocystis carinii*. J Infect Dis 154:315-322, 1986.

241. Leoung GS, Mills J, Hopewell PC, Hughes W, Wofsy C. Dapsone-trimethoprim for *Pneumocystis carinii* pneumonia

in the acquired immunodeficiency syndrome. Ann Intern Med 105:45-48, 1986.

242. Hughes WT, Williams B, Williams B, Pearson T. The nosocomial colonization of T Bear. Infect Control 7:495-500, 1986.

243. Hughes WT. Pneumocystis pneumonia. In: Rudolph A, ed. Pediatrics. 18th ed. East Norwalk: Appleton-Century-Crofts, pp 692-693, 1987.

244. Hughes WT. Infection of immunosuppressed host. In: Rudolph A, ed. Pediatrics. 18th ed. East Norwalk: Appleton-Century-Crofts, pp 473-475, 1987.

245. Hughes WT. *Candidiasis*. In: Feigin R, Cherry J, eds. Textbook of pediatric infectious diseases. 2nd ed. Philadelphia: WB Saunders Co, pp 1939-1949, 1987.

246. Anderson DC, Hughes WT. *Pneumocystis carinii* pneumonia. In: Feigin R, Cherry J, eds. Textbook of pediatric infectious diseases. 2nd ed. Philadelphia: WB Saunders Co, pp 319-327, 1987.

247. Hughes WT. *Pneumocystis carinii* pneumonia. Boca Raton: CRC Press, Vol I, pp 131 and Vol II, pp 136, 1987.

248. Hughes WT. Sulfonamides and trimethoprim. In: Peterson PK, Verhoef J, eds. The antimicrobial agents annual II. Amsterdam: Elsevier Science Pub, pp 204-211, 1987.

249. Stokes DC, Gigliotti F, Rehg JE, Snellgrove RL, Hughes WT. Experimental *Pneumocystis carinii* pneumonia in the ferret. Br J Exp Pathol 68:267-276, 1987.

250. Aronoff SC, Hughes WT, Kohl S, Speck WT, Wald ER. Advances in pediatric infectious diseases. Vol 2. Yearbook Medical Pub, 1987.

251. Hughes WT, Rivera GK, Schell MJ, Thornton D, Lott L. Successful intermittent chemoprophylaxis for *Pneumocystis carinii* pneumonitis. N Engl J Med 316:1627-1632, 1987.

252. Hughes WT. *Pneumocystis carinii*. In: Weatherall J, Ledingham JGG, Warrell DA, eds. Oxford textbook of medicine. 2nd ed. Oxford Medical Publication, pp 5.504-5.506, 1987.

253. Hughes WT. Pneumonia in the immunocompromised child. Semin Respir Infect 2:177-183, 1987.

254. Hughes WT. Treatment and prophylaxis for *Pneumocystis carinii* pneumonia. Parasitology Today 3:332-335, 1987.

255. Hughes WT. *Pneumocystis carinii* pneumonitis (Editorial). N Engl J Med 317:1021-1023, 1987.

256. Hughes WT. Persistent thrush in young infants (Letter discussion). Pediatr Infect Dis 6:1075, 1987.

257. Hughes WT. Aspergillosis. In: Nelson J, ed. Current therapy in pediatric infectious disease. Philadelphia: DC Decker Inc, pp 164-165, 1988.

258. Hughes WT, Gigliotti F. Nomenclature for *Pneumocystis carinii*. J Infect Dis 157:432-433, 1988.

259. Aronoff SG, Hughes WT, Kohl S, Speck W, Wald ER. Advances in pediatric infectious diseases. Vol 3. Yearbook Medical Pub, 1988.

260. Laraya-Cuasay L, Hughes WT. Interstitial lung diseases in children. Vol I, 194 pp; Vol II, 201 pp; Vol III, 188 pp. Boca Raton: CRC Press, 1988.

261. Hughes WT. A tribute to toilet paper. Rev Infect Dis 10:218-222, 1988.

262. Stokes DC, Shenep JL, Horowitz ME, Hughes WT. Presentation of *Pneumocystis carinii* pneumonia as unilateral hyperlucent lung. Chest 94:201-202, 1988.

263. Hughes WT. Sulfonamides and trimethoprim. In: Peterson PK, Verhoef J eds. The antimicrobial agents annual 3. Chapter 18. Amsterdam: Elsevier Science Pub, pp 229-237, 1988.

264. Gigliotti F, Hughes WT. Passive immunoprophylaxis with specified monoclonal antibody confers partial protection against *Pneumocystis carinii* pneumonitis in animal models. J Clin Invest 81:1666-1668, 1988.

265. Hughes WT. Comparison of dosages, intervals and drugs in the prevention of *Pneumocystis carinii* pneumonia. Antimicrob Agents Chemother 32:623-625, 1988.

266. Hughes WT. Treatment of *Pneumocystis carinii* pneumonia in AIDS (Letter). N Engl J Med 318:990, 1988.

267. Mills J, Leoung G, Medina I, Hopewell PC, Hughes WT, Wofsy C. Dapsone treatment of *Pneumocystis carinii* pneumonia in the acquired immunodeficiency syndrome. Antimicrob Agents Chemother 32:1057-1060, 1988.

268. Gigliotti F, Ballou LR, Hughes WT, Mosley B. Purification and initial characterization of ferret *P. carinii* surface antigen

capable of inducing protective antibody. J Infect Dis 158:848-854, 1988.

269. Leggiadro R, Barrett FF, Hughes WT. Disseminated histoplasmosis of infancy. Pediatr Infect Dis J 7:799-805, 1988.

270. Shenep SL, Hughes WT, Roberson PK, Blankenship KR, Baker D, Meyer WH, Gigliotti F, Sixbey J, Santana V, Feldman S, Lott L. Decreased incidence of breakthrough bacteremia with vancomycin, ticarcillin and amikacin versus ticarcillin-clavulanate and amikacin in febrile, neutropenic children with cancer. N Engl J Med 319:1053, 1988.

271. Wang WC, Parham DM, Herrod HG, Hughes WT. An unusual chronic maculopapular rash associated with human immunodeficiency virus infection. South Med J 82:386-389, 1989.

272. Hughes WT. Animal models for *Pneumocystis carinii* pneumonia. J Protozool 36:41-45, 1989.

273. Hughes WT. Pneumocystosis. In: Goldsmith RS, Heyneman D, eds. Tropical medicine and parasitology. Norwalk: Appleton and Lange, pp 329-332, 1989.

274. Hughes WT. *Pneumocystis carinii*: taxing taxonomy. Eur J Epidemiol 5:265-270, 1989.

275. Aronoff SG, Hughes WT, Kohl S, Speck W, Wald ER. In: Advances in pediatric infectious diseases. Vol 4. Yearbook Medical Pub, 1989.

276. Hughes WT. Antibiotics for the treatment of febrile children with neutropenia and cancer. Correspondence - Reply - N Engl J Med 320:939, 1989.

277. Hughes WT. Nomenclature for *Pneumocystis carinii* - Reply - J Infect Dis 159:366, 1989.

278. Hughes WT. Aspergillosis. In: Oski F, ed. Principles and practice of pediatrics. JB Lippincott Co, pp 1255-1256, 1990.

279. Hughes WT. The dermatophytoses. In: Oski F, ed. Principles and practice of pediatrics. JB Lippincott Co, pp 1254-1255, 1990.

280. Hughes WT. Candidiasis. In: Oski F, ed. Principles and practice of pediatrics. JB Lippincott Co, pp 1251-1253, 1990.

281. Hughes WT. Cryptosporidiosis. In: Oski F, ed. Principles and practice of pediatrics. JB Lippincott Co, pp 1271-1272, 1990.

282. Hughes WT. *Pneumocystis carinii*: advances in biology, prophylaxis and treatment. In: McAdam KPWJ, ed. New strategies in parasitology. London: Churchill Livingstone, pp 276-287, 1990.

283. Hughes WT, Gray VL, Gutteridge WE, Latter VS, Pudney M. Efficacy of a hydroxynaphthoquinone, 566C80, in experimental *Pneumocystis carinii* pneumonitis. Antimicrob Agents Chemother 34:225-228, 1990.

284. Hughes WT. Empiric antimicrobial therapy in the febrile granulocytopenic patient. Infect Control Hosp Epidemiol 11:151-156, 1990.

285. Hughes W. Weekly dapsone for prophylaxis of *Pneumocystis carinii* pneumonitis. Nurse Stand 5(8): 16, Nov. 1992.

286. Hughes W, Armstrong D, Bodey GP, Feld R, Mandell GL, Meyers JD, Pizzo PA, Shenep JL, Schimpff SC, Wade JC, Young

LS, Yow MD. Guidelines for the use of antimicrobial agents in neutropenic patients with unexplained fever: a statement by the Infection Review Society of America. J Infect Dis 161:381-396, 1990.

287. Hughes WT. *Pneumocystis carinii* pneumonitis. In: Chernick V, Kendig EL, eds. Disorders of the respiratory tract in children. 5th ed. Philadelphia: WB Saunders Co, pp 381-388, 1990.

288. Hughes WT. Histoplasmosis. In: Chernick V, Kendig EL, eds. Disorders of the respiratory tract in children. 5th ed. Philadelphia: WB Saunders Co, pp 781-787, 1990.

289. Hughes WT. Oncology and hematology. In: Moxon R, Sect ed. Current opinion in pediatrics. Curr Sci 2:110-112, 1990.

290. Hughes WT. The prevention of *Pneumocystis carinii* pneumonia. Hosp Pract 25:33-43, 1990.

291. Hughes WT. Tularemia. In: Gellis S, Kagan B eds. Current pediatric therapy. 13th ed. Philadelphia: WB Saunders Co, pp 537-538, 1990.

292. Hughes WT. *Pneumocystis carinii* pneumonitis. In: Gellis S, Kagan B, eds. Current pediatric therapy. 13th ed. Philadelphia: WB Saunders Co, pp 553-555, 1990.

293. Flynn PM, Magill HL, Jenkins JJ, Pearson T, Crist WM and Hughes WT. Aspergillus osteomyelitis in a child treated for acute lymphoblastic leukemia. Pediatr Infect Dis J 9:733-736, 1990.

294. Hughes WT. "The article reviewed" (Commentary). Oncology 4:53-54, 1990.

295. Aronoff SG, Hughes WT, Kohl S, Speck W, Wald ER. In: Advances in pediatric infectious diseases. Vol 5. Yearbook Medical Pub, 1990.

296. Hughes WT, Kennedy W, Dugdale M, Land MA, Stein DS, Weems JJ Jr, Palte S, Lancaster D, Kovnar SG, Morrison RE. Prevention of *Pneumocystis carinii* pneumonitis in AIDS patients with weekly dapsone. Lancet 336:1066, 1990.

297. Hughes WT. Infections in the immunosuppressed host. In: Summit RL, ed. Comprehensive Pediatrics. St. Louis: CV Mosby Co, pp 891-895, 1990.

298. Vargas S, Hughes WT, Giannini MA. Aspergillus in pepper. Lancet 336:881, 1990.

299. Hughes WT. Enteroviral infections. In: Summit RL, ed. Comprehensive Pediatrics. St. Louis: CV Mosby Co, pp 858-861, 1990.

300. Hughes WT. Mycotic diseases. In: Summit RL, ed. Comprehensive Pediatrics. St. Louis: CV Mosby Co, pp 881-886, 1990.

301. Hughes WT. *Pneumocystis carinii* pneumonia. In: Pizzo P, Wilfert C, eds. Pediatric AIDS: The challenge of HIV infection in infants, children and adolescents. Baltimore: Williams & Williams, pp 288-298, 1991.

302. Hughes WT. Prevention and treatment of *Pneumocystis carinii* pneumonitis. In: Ann Rev Medicine. Vol. 42. Palo Alto: Annual Review Inc, pp 287-295, 1991.

303. Hughes WT, Parham DM. Molluscum contagiosum in children with cancer or AIDS. Pediatr Infect Dis J 10:152-156, 1991.

304. Shenep JL, Hughes WT, Flynn PM, Crawford R. An anonymous, encrypted registry for pediatric patients with human immunodeficiency virus infection. Pediatr AIDS/HIV Infect:Fetus to Adolescent 2:16-23, 1991.

305. Aronoff SG, Hughes WT, Kohn S, Speck W, Wald ER. In: Advances in pediatric infectious diseases. Vol 6. Yearbook Medical Pub, 1991.

306. Hughes WT. Pneumocystosis. In: Strickland GT, ed. Hunter's tropical medicine. 7th ed. Philadelphia: WB Saunders Co, pp 670-672, 1991.

307. Hughes WT. *Pneumocystis carinii*. In: Barron S, ed. Medical microbiology. 3rd ed. Churchill Livingstone, pp 1059-1063, 1991.

308. Hughes WT. Infection of immunosuppressed host. In: Rudolph A, ed. Pediatrics. 19th ed. Appleton and Lange, pp 543-545, 1991.

309. Hughes WT. Pneumocystis pneumonia. In: Rudolph A, ed. Pediatrics. 19th ed. Appleton and Lange, pp 774-775, 1991.

310. Hughes WT. Treatment of established bacterial and fungal infections in patients with hematologic malignancy. In: Wiernick PH, *et al*, eds. Neoplastic disease of blood. 2nd ed. New York: Churchill Livingstone, pp 805-816, 1991.

311. Kavanagh K, Hughes WT, Parham D, Chanin LR. Fungal sinusitis in immunocompromised children with neoplasms. Ann Otol Rhinol Laryngol 100:331-336, 1991.

312. Hughes WT, Kennedy W, Shenep JL, Flynn PM, Hetherington SV, Fullen G, Lancaster DJ, Stein DS, Palte S, Rosenbaum D,

Liao SHT, Blum R, Rogers M. Safety and pharmacokinetics of 566C80, a hydroxynaphthoquinone with anti-*Pneumocystis carinii* activity: A phase I study in HIV-infected men. J Infect Dis 163:843-848, 1991.

313. Hughes WT. *Pneumocystis carinii* pneumonia: New approaches to diagnosis, treatment and prevention. Pediatr Infect Dis J 10:391-399, 1991.

314. Hughes WT, Killmar J. Synergistic anti-*Pneumocystis carinii* effects of erythromycin and sulfisoxazole. J AIDS 4:532-537, 1991.

315. Shenep JL, Adair JR, Hughes WT, Roberson PK, Flynn PM, Brodkey TO, Fullen GH, Kennedy WT, Oakes LL, Marina NM. Infrared, thermistor, and glass-mercury thermometry for measurement of body temperature in children with cancer. Clin Pediatr (Suppl) 36-41, April 1991.

316. Marina NM, Flynn PM, Rivera GK, Hughes WT. *Candida tropicalis* and *Candida albicans* fungemia in children with leukemia. Cancer 68:594-599, 1991.

317. Hughes WT. Neumonia por *Pneumocystic carinii*: nuevos metodos do diagnostico, tratamiento y prevencion. MTA Pediatria 12:428-450, 1991.

318. Langhon BE, Allandeen HS, Becker JM, Current WL, Feinberg J, Frenkel JK, Hafner R, Hughes WT, Laughlin CA, Myers JD, Schrager LK, Young LS. Summary of the Workshop on Future Directions in Discovery and Development of Therapeutic Agents for Opportunistic Infections Associated with AIDS. National Institutes of Health. J Infect Dis 164:244-251, 1991.

319. Leggiadro RJ, Kline MW, Hughes WT. Extrapulmonary crypto-coccosis in children with AIDS. Pediatr Infect Dis J 10:658-662, 1991.

320. Hinds P, Wentz, Hughes W, Pearson T, Sims A, Mason B, Pratt M, Austin B. An investigation of safety of the blood reinfusion step used with Hickman catheters in children with cancer. J Pediatr Oncol Nur 8:159-164, 1991.

321. Falloon J, Kovacs V, Hughes W, O'Neill D, Polis M, Davey R, Rogers M, LaFon S, Feuerstein I, Lancaster D, Land M, Tuazon C, Dohn M, Greenberg S, Lane HC, Masur H. A preliminary evaluation of 566C80 for the treatment of *Pneumocystis* pneumonia in patients with the acquired immunodeficiency syndrome. N Engl J Med 325:1534-1538, 1991.

322. Hughes WT. Closing comments: *Pneumocystis carinii*. J Protozol 38:S243, 1991.

323. Hughes WT. *Pneumocystis carinii*: from Bristol to Bozeman. J Protozol 38:52, 1991.

324. Hughes WT, Armstrong D, Bodey GP, Feld R, Mandell GL, Meyers JD, Pizzo PA, Schimpff SC, Shenep JL, Wade JC, Young LS, Flynn PM. (Correspondence – Reply) J Infect Dis 163:202-203, 1991.

325. Hughes WT. Macrolide-antifol synergism in anti-*Pneumocystis carinii* therapeutics. J Protozol 38:160S, 1991.

326. Hughes WT. Guidelines for the use of antimicrobial agents in neutropenic patients with unexplained fever. Correspondence - Reply - J Infect Dis 163:201, 1991.

327. Hughes WT. Forward. In: Hopkin JM. *Pneumocystis carinii*. Oxford University Press, Oxford, 1991.

328. Aronoff S, Hughes WT, Kohl S, Speck W, Wald E. Advances in pediatric infectious diseases. Vol. 7. St. Louis: Mosby Yearbook, 1992.

329. Hughes WT. Prevention of *Pneumocystis carinii* pneumonia. Infect Med 9:11-14, 1992.

330. Hughes WT. Commentary: *Pneumocystis carinii* infection: An update. In: Williams & Wilkins. Classics in Medicine 71:175-178, 1992.

331. Hughes WT. Prevention of infection in the neutropenic patient. In: Patrick C, ed. Infections in immunocomprised infants and children. New York: Churchill Livingstone, Inc, pp 771-784, 1992.

332. Hughes WT. *Pneumocystis carinii*. In: Gorbach S, Bartlett J, Blacklow N, eds. Infectious diseases. Philadelphia: WB Saunders Co, pp 1994-1996, 1992.

333. Hughes WT. Malnutrition. In: Patrick C, ed. Infections in immunocomprised infants and children. New York: Churchill Livingstone, Inc, pp 329-333, 1992.

334. Hughes WT. *Pneumocystis carinii* pneumonia. In: Gorbach S, Bartlett J, Blacklow N, eds. Infectious diseases. Philadelphia: WB Saunders Co, pp 494-497, 1992.

335. Hughes WT. Cryptococcosis. In: Patrick C, ed. Infections in immunocompromised infants and children. New York: Churchill Livingstone, Inc, pp 551-556, 1992.

336. Hughes WT. *Pneumocystis carinii* pneumonia. In, Patrick C, ed. Infections in immunocompromised infants and children. New York: Churchill Livingstone, Inc, pp 711-718, 1992.

337. Leggiadro RJ, Barrett FF, Hughes WT. Extrapulmonary crypto-coccosis in immunocompromised infants and children. Pediatr Infect Dis J 11:43-47, 1992.

338. Hughes WR, Pizzo PA, Wade JC, Armstrong D, Webb CD, Young LS. General guidelines for the evaluation of new anti-infective agents for the treatment of febrile episodes in neutropenic patients. Evaluation of new anti-infective drugs for the treatment of febrile episodes in neutropenic patients. C I D (Suppl) 15:206-215, November 1992.

339. Hughes WT. New drugs for infections in patients with cancer. Cancer (Suppl) 70:959-965, August 15, 1992.

340. Hughes WT, Anderson DC. *Pneumocystis carinii* pneumonia. In: Feigin RD, Cherry JD, eds. Textbook of Pediatric Infectious Diseases. 3rd ed. Philadelphia: WB Saunders, pp 289-297, 1992.

341. Hughes WT. A new drug (566C80) for the treatment of *Pneumocystis carinii* pneumonitis (editorial). Ann Intern Med 116:953-954, June 1992.

342. Hughes WT. Candidiasis. In: Feigin RD, Cherry JD, eds. Textbook of Pediatric Infectious Diseases. 3rd ed. Philadelphia: WB Saunders, pp 1907-1916, 1992.

343. Hughes WT. New drug offers alternative treatment for PCP (Medigrams). Am Fam Physician 46:1257-1258, October 1992.

344. Hughes WT. *Pneumocystis carinii* pneumonia: treatment and prevention. IDN 11:81-84, November 1992.

345. Flynn PM, Hughes WT. Infections in immunocompromised children. In: Voûte PA, Barrett A, Lemerle J, eds. Cancer in children. 3rd ed. Springer-Verlag, Berlin, 1992, pp 59-70.

346. Hughes WT. Prevention of infections in patients with T-Cell defects. C I D 17:(S-2)368-372, 1993.

347. Aronoff SC, Hughes WT, Kohl S, Speck WT, Wald ER, eds. Adv Pediatr Infect Dis 8:214, 1993.

348. Vargas SL, Patrick CC, Ayers GD, Hughes WT. Modulating effect of dietary carbohydrate supplementation on *Candida albicans* colonization and invasion in a neutropenic mouse model. Infect Immun 61:619-626, February 1993.

349. Hughes WT. Tularemia. In: Burg FD, Inglefinger JH, Wald ER, eds. Current pediatric therapy. 14th ed. WB Saunders, pp 579-580, 1993.

350. Hughes WT. Pneumonia in the immunosuppressed host. In: Hilman BC, ed. Pediatric respiratory disease. Philadelphia: WB Saunders, pp 296-304, 1993.

351. Hughes WT, Leoung G, Kramer F, Bozzette S, Safrin S, Frame P, Clumeck N, Masur H, Lancaster D, Chan C, Lavelle J, Rosenstock J, Falloon J, Feinberg J, LaFon S, Rogers M, Sattler F. Comparison of atovaquone (566C80) with trimethoprim-sulfamethoxazole for the treatment of *Pneumocystis carinii* pneumonia in patients with AIDS. N Engl J Med 328:1521-1527, 1993.

352. Hughes WT, Jacobus DP, Canfield C, Killmar J. Anti-*Pneumocystis carinii* activity of PS-15, a new biguanide folate antagonist. Antimicrob Agents Chemother 37:1417-1419, 1993.

353. Vargas SL, Shenep JL, Flynn PM, Pui C-H, Santana VM, Hughes WT. Azithromycin for treatment of severe *Cryptosporidium* diarrhea in two children with cancer. J Pediatr 123:154-156, 1993.

354. Hughes WT. *Pneumocystis carinii* pneumonitis. In: Burg FD, Inglefinger JR, Wald ER, eds. Current Pediatric Therapy. 14th ed. pp 593-595, 1993.

355. Flynn PM, Marina NM, Rivera GK, Hughes WT. Candida tropicalis infection in children with leukemia. Leuk Lymphoma 10:369-376, 1993.

356. Hughes WT. *Pneumocystis carinii* pneumonia. In: Pizzo P, Wilfert C, eds. Pediatric AIDS: The challenge of HIV infection in infants, children and adolescents. 2nd ed. Baltimore: Williams and Wilkins, pp 405-416, 1994.

357. Hughes WT. Opportunistic infections in children with human immunodeficiency virus infection. Pediatric HIV Forum 2:1-5, 1994.

358. Hughes WT. Opportunistic infections in AIDS patients: Current management and prevention. Postgraduate Medicine 95:81-93, 1994.

359. Sanyal SK, Chebib FS, Gilbert R, Hughes WT. Sequential changes in vital signs and acid-base and blood-gas profiles in *Pneumocystis carinii* pneumonia in children with cancer: basis for a scoring system to identify patients who will require ventilatory support. Am J Respir Crit Care Med 149:1092-1098, 1994.

360. Hughes WT, Hutcheson RH, Gallemore GH, Higgs BC, Chesney PJ, Clifford RR, Jr. Statement of the Committee on Infectious Diseases, Tennessee Chapter, American Academy of Pediatrics. J Tenn Med Assoc :21, 1994.

361. Hughes WT. Candidiasis. In: Oski F, ed. Principles and practice of pediatrics. 2nd ed. Philadelphia: JB Lippincott Co, pp 1369-1370, 1994.

362. Hughes WT. The Dermathophytoses. In: Oski F, ed. Principles and practice of pediatrics. 2nd ed. Philadelphia: JB Lippincott Co, pp 1371-1372, 1994.

363. Hughes WT. Aspergillosis. In: Oski F, ed. Principles and practice of pediatrics. 2nd ed. Philadelphia: JB Lippincott Co, pp 1372-1374, 1994.

364. Hughes WT. Cryptosporidiosis. In: Oski F, ed. Principles and practice of pediatrics. 2nd ed. Philadelphia: JB Lippincott Co, pp 1389-1390, 1994.

365. Aronoff SC, Hughes WT, Kohl S, Speck WT, Wald ER, eds. Adv Pediatr Infect Dis 9:266, 1994.

366. Hughes W, Killmar J, Oz H. Relative potency of ten drugs with anti-*Pneumocystis carinii* activity in an animal model. J Infect Dis 170:906-911, 1994.

367. Shenep JL, Hughes WT, Flynn PM, Robertson PK, Behm FG, Fullen GH, Kovnar SG, Guito KP, Brodkey TO. Decreased counts of blood neutrophils, monocytes and platelets in human immunodeficiency virus-infected children and adults treated with diethyldithio-carbamate. Antimicrob Agents Chemother 38:1644-1646, 1994.

368. Pui C-H, Hughes WT, Evans WE, Crist WM. Correspondence - Prevention of *Pneumocystis carinii* pneumonia in children with cancer. J Clin Oncol 12:1522-1525, 1994.

369. Hughes WT. Pneumocystis carinii: What is it and from whence does it come? J Eukaryotic Microb 41:123S, 1994.

370. Wakefield AE, Fritscher CC, Malin AS, Gwanzura L, Hughes WT, Miller RF. Genetic diversity in human-derived *Pneumocystis carinii* isolates from four geographical locations shown by analysis of mitochondrial rRNA gene sequences. J Clin Microbiol 32:2959-2961, 1994.

371. Hughes WT. Hydroxynaphthoquinones. In: Walzer P. *Pneumocystis carinii* pneumonia. 2nd ed. New York: Marcel Dekker Inc, pp 603-614, 1994.

372. Hughes WT. Clinical manifestations in children. In: Walzer P. *Pneumocystis carinii* pneumonia. New York: Marcel Dekker Inc, pp 319-329, 1994.

373. Hughes WT. New drugs for the prevention and treatment of *Pneumocystis carinii* pneumonia. In: Büchner, et al, eds. Acute Leukemias IV: Prognostic Factors. Springer-Verlag, Berlin, Heidelberg pp 735-737, 1994.

374. Hughes WT. The role of atovaquone tablet in treating *Pneumocystis carinii* pneumonia. J Acquir Immune Defic Syndr 8:247-252, 1995.

375. Hughes WT. Billy Andrews: a unique individual. J Perinatology 15:102, 1995.

376. Hughes WT. carinii (original article). Yearbook of science and technology. New York: McGraw-Hill, pp 268-270, 1995.

377. Hughes WT, LaFon S, Masur H. Adverse events associated with trimethoprim-sulfamethoxazole and atovaquone during the

treatment of AIDS related Pneumocystis pneumonia. J Infect Dis 171:1295-1301, 1995.

378. Hughes WT. Pneumocystis carinii pneumonia. The Report on Pediatric Infectious Diseases. Churchill Livingstone Co, vol 5, pp 19-20, 1995.

379. Flynn PM, Shenep JL, Crawford R, Hughes WT. Use of abdominal computed tomography for identifying disseminated fungal infection in pediatric cancer patients. Clin Infect Dis 20:964-970, 1995.

380. Vargas SL, Hughes WT, Wakefield AE, Oz H. Limited persistence and subsequent elimination of *Pneumocystis carinii* from the lungs after *P. carinii* pneumonia. J Infect Dis 172:506-510, 1995.

381. Hughes WT, Oz HS. Successful prevention and treatment of babesiosis with atovaquone. J Infect Dis 172:1042-1046, 1995.

382. Hughes WT. *Pneumocystis carinii* infections in mother, infants and in non-AIDS elderly adults. In: Sattler F, Walzer P, eds. *Pneumocystis carinii*. Baillière's Clinical Infectious Diseases. Baillière Tindall, London, pp 461-470, 1995.

383. Hughes WT. Pneumocystis in infants and children (letter). N Engl J Med 333:320-321, 1995.

384. Simonds RJ, Hughes WT, Feinberg J, Nevin TR. Preventing *Pneumocystis carinii* pneumonia in persons infected with human immunodeficiency virus. Clin Infect Dis 21 (Suppl):S44-48, 1995.

385. Aronoff SC, Hughes WT, Kohl S, Speck WT, Wald ER. Advance in Pediatric Infectious Diseases, vol 10, 1995.

386. Hughes WT. Postulates for the evaluation of adverse reactions to drugs. Clin Infect Dis 20:179-182, 1995.

387. Hughes WT. The Eye. In: Taeusch NW, Christiansen R, Buescher ES, eds. Pediatric and neonatal tests and procedures. WB Saunders, pp 421-426, 1995.

388. Hughes WT. Fluid and metabolic therapy. In: Taeusch NW, et al, eds. Pediatric and neonatal tests and procedures. WB Saunders, pp 253-294, 1995.

389. Hughes WT. *Pneumocystis carinii* pneumonitis. In: Burg FD, Inglefinger JR, Wald ER, eds. Current Pediatric Therapy, 15th ed. WB Saunders, pp 687-689, 1996.

390. Aronoff SC, Hughes WT, Kohl S, Speck WT, Wald ER. Advances in Pediatric Infectious Diseases, vol 11, pp 489, 1996.

391. Hughes WT. Recent advances in the prevention of *Pneumocystis carinii* pneumonia. Advances in Pediatr Infect Dis 11:163-186, 1996.

392. Hughes WT, Flynn PM, Williams B. Nosocomial infection in patients with neoplastic disease. In: Mayhall CG, ed. Hospital Epidemiology and Infection Control, Williams and Wilkins Co, pp 618-631, 1996.

393. Hughes WT. *Pneumocystis carinii* pneumonitis. In: Behrman RF, Kliegman R, Arvin DM, eds. Nelson textbook of pediatrics. 15th ed, WB Saunders Co, pp 951-952, 1996.

394. Hughes WT. Infections in the compromised host. In: Behrman RF, Kliegman R, Arvin DM, eds. Nelson textbook of pediatrics. 15th ed, WB Saunders Co, pp 733-744, 1996.

395. Hughes WT. Treatment of established bacterial and fungal infections in patients with hematologic malignancy. In: Wiernik PH, Canellos GP, Dutcher JP, Kyle RA. Neoplastic diseases of the blood, 3rd ed. Churchill Livingstone, pp 1027-1040, 1996.

396. Hughes WT, Killmar J. Monodrug efficacy of sulfonamides in prophylaxis for *Pneumocystis carinii* pneumonia. Antimicrob Agents Chemother 40:962-965, 1996.

397. Oz HS, Hughes WT, Vargas SL. Search for extrapulmonary *Pneumocystis carinii* in an animal model. J Parasitol 82(2):357-359, 1996.

398. Oz HS, Hughes WT. Effect of gender and dexamethasone dose on the experimental host for *Pneumocystis carinii*. Lab Anim Sci 46:109-110, 1996.

399. Hughes WT. *Pneumocystis* pneumonia. In: Rudolph A, ed. Pediatrics, 20th ed. Appleton & Lange, pp 775-777, 1996.

400. Hughes WT. Infection of the immunosuppressed host. In: Rudolph A, ed. Pediatrics. 20th ed. Appleton and Lange, pp 517-519, 1996.

401. Hughes WT. Pneumocystis carinii. In: Schlossberg D. Current therapy for infectious disease. Mosby-Year Book, pp 570-571, 1996.

402. Oz H, Hughes WT. Acute fulminating babesiosis in hamsters infected with *Babesia microti*. Int J Parasitol 26:667-770, 1996.

403. Hughes WT. *Pneumocystis carinii*. In: Baron S, ed. Medical Microbiology: General Concepts Study Guide, 4th ed. University of Texas Medical Branch, Galveston, Pub, p 233, 1996.

404. Hughes WT. *Pneumocystis carinii*. In: Baron S. Medical microbiology, 4th ed. University of Texas Medical Branch, Galveston, Pub., pp 1019-1022, 1996.

405. Hughes WT. *Pneumocystis carinii* pneumonia in cancer patients. Infect Med 13:857-867, 1996.

406. Hughes WT. Opportunistic infections in children. Hong Kong J Pediatr 1:100-104, 1996.

407. Hughes WT. *Helicobacter pylori* infection. Pediatr Ann 25:491-493, 1996.

408. Hughes WT. Pneumocystis carinii. In: Long SS, Pinkering L, Prober C, eds. Principles and Practice of Pediatric Infectious Diseases. Churchill Livingstone, pp 1417-1420, 1997.

409. Oz H, Hughes WT. Novel *anti-Pneumocystis carinii* effects of the immunosuppressant mycophenolate mofetil in contrast to provocative effects of tacrolimus, sirolimus and dexamethasone. J Infect Dis 175:901-904, 1997.

410. Oz H, Hughes WT, Rehg J. Efficacy of lasalocid against murine *Pneumocystis carinii* pneumonitis. Antimicrob Agents Chemother 41:191-192, 1997.

411. Hughes WT. *Pneumocystis carinii* pneumonia. In: Kassirer J, Greene HL, eds. Current Therapy in Adult Medicine, 4th Ed. Philadelphia: Mosby Yearbook, Inc, pp 336-337, 1997.

412. Oz H, Hughes WT. *Pneumocystis carinii* infection alters GTP-binding sites in lungs. J Parasitol 83:679-685, 1997.

413. Hughes WT. The athlete: An immunocompromised host. Adv Pediatr Infect Res 13:79-99, 1997.

414. Pui C-H, Boyett JM, Hughes WT, Rivera GK, Hancock ML, Sandlund T, Synold T, Relling MV, Ribeiro RC, Crist WM, Evans WE. Human granulocyte colony-stimulating factor after induction chemotherapy in children with acute lymphocytic leukemia. N Engl J Med 336:1781-1787, 1997.

415. Hughes WT, Armstrong D, Bodey GP, Brown AE, Edwards JE, Feld R, Pizzo P, Rolston KVI, Shenep JL, Young LS. 1997 Guidelines for the use of antimicrobial agents in neutropenic patients with unexplained fever. C.I.D. 25:551-573, 1997.

416. Hughes WT. *Pneumocystis carinii* pneumonia. Infectious Diseases in Clinical Practice 6:379-384, 1997.

417. Aronoff SC, Hughes WT, Kohl S, Prince A, Wald ER. Advances in Pediatric Infectious Diseases, vol 13, 389 pp, St. Louis: Mosby, 1997.

417. Hughes WT. *Pneumocystis carinii*. Current Therapy in Internal Medicine, 4th ed. Mosby-Yearbook Inc, St. Louis, pp 336-337, 1997.

418. Hughes WT, Anderson DC. *Pneumocystis carinii* pneumonia. In: Feigin RD, Cherry JD, eds. Textbook of pediatric infectious diseases, 4th ed. Philadelphia: WB Saunders Co, pp 2490-2498, 1998.

419. Hughes WT, Flynn PM. Candidiasis. In: Feigin RD, Cherry JD, eds. Textbook of pediatric infectious diseases, 4th ed. Philadelphia: WB Saunders Co, pp 2303-2313, 1998.

420. Hughes WT. Cryptococcosis. In: Feigin RD, Cherry JD, eds. Textbook of pediatric infectious diseases, 4th ed. Philadelphia: WB Saunders Co, pp 2332-2337, 1998.

421. Choueiry MA, Scurto PL, Flynn PM, Rao BN, Hughes WT. Disseminated infection with *Mycobacterium fortuitum* in a patient with desmoid tumor. C.I.D. 26:238-238, 1998.

422. Hughes WT. Commentary on abacavir. Drugs 55(5):737-738, 1998.

423. Hughes WT. *Pneumocystis carinii* pneumonia. In: Chernick V, Boat TF, eds. Kendig's Disorders of the Respiratory Tract in Children, 6th ed. WB Saunders Co, Philadelphia, pp 503-511, 1998.

424. Flynn PM, Hughes WT. Histoplasmosis. In: Chernick V, Boat TF, eds. Kendig's Disorders of the Respiratory Tract in Children, 6th ed. WB Saunders Co, Philadelphia, pp 946-953, 1998.

425. Hughes WT. *Pneumocystis carinii* pneumonia. In: Gorbach SL, Bartlett JG, Blasklow NR, eds. Infectious diseases, 2nd ed. WB Saunders Co, Chapter 59, pp 601-604.

426. Hughes WT. *Pneumocystis carinii*. In: Gorbach SL, Bartlett JG, Blasklow NR, eds. Infectious diseases, 2nd ed. WB Saunders Co, Chapter 291, pp 2440-2441, 1998.

427. Hughes WT. Current issues in the epidemiology, transmission and reactivation of *Pneumocystis carinii*. Semin Respir Infect 13:283-288, 1998.

428. Al-Moshen I, Hughes WT. Systemic antifungal therapy: Past, present and future. Ann Saudi Med 18:28-38, 1998.

429. Hughes WT, Silos EM, La Fron S, Rogers M, Woolley JL, Davis C, Studenberg S, Pattishall E, Freeze T, Snyder G, Staton S. Effects of aerosolized synthetic surfactant, atovaquone and the combination of these on murine *Pneumocystis carinii* pneumonia. J Infect Dis 177:1046-1056, 1998.

430. Hughes WT. The use of dapsone in the prevention and treatment of *Pneumocystis carinii* pneumonia: A review. Clin Infect Dis 27:191-204, 1998.

431. Hughes WT. Prologue to AIDS: The recognition of infectious opportunists. Medicine 77:227-232, 1998.

432. Hughes WT. Commentary on Amprenavir. Drugs 55:844, 1998.

433. Hughes W, Dorenbaum A, Yogev R, Beauchamp B, Xu J, McNamara J, Moye J, Purdue L, van Dyke R, Rogers M, Sadler B. A phase I safety and pharmacokinetics study of micronized atovaquone in human immunodeficiency virus (HIV)-infected infants and children. Antimicrob Agents Chemother 42:1315-1318, 1998.

434. Hughes WT. Guidelines for the use of antimicrobial agents in neutropenic patients with unexplained fever. Infect Oncol 2:1-7, 1998.

435. Aronoff SC, Hughes WT, Kohl S, Prince A. Adv Pediatr Infect Dis 14:301, 1998.

436. Hughes WT. *Cryptococcus neoformans*. In: Brug FD, Ingelfinger JR, Wald ER, Polin RA, eds. Current Pediatric Therapy, 16th ed. WB Saunders Co, Philadelphia, p 148, 1999.

437. Hughes WT. Candidiasis. In: DeAngelis CD, et al. Oski's Pediatrics: Principles and Practice, 3rd ed. Lippincott-Raven, pp 1151-1153, 1999.

438. Hughes WT. Cryptosporidiosis. In: DeAngelis CD, et al. Oski's Pediatrics: Principles and Practice, 3rd ed. Lippincott-Raven, pp 1174-1176, 1999.

439. Hughes WT. Aspergillosis. In: DeAngelis CD, et al. Oski's Pediatrics: Principles and Practice, 3rd ed. Lippincott-Raven, pp 1155-1157, 1999.

440. Hughes WT. Infectious Complications. In: Pui C-H, ed. Childhood Leukemia. Cambridge University Press, pp 482-499, 1999.

441. Hughes W, McDowell JA, Shenep J, Flynn P, Kline MW, Yogev R, Symonds W, Lou Y, Hetherington S. Safety and single-dose pharmacokinetics of abacavir (1592U89) in human immuno-deficiency virus type 1-infected children. Antimicrob Agents Chemother 43:609-615, 1999.

442. Oz HS, Hughes WT, Rehg JE. Rat model for dual opportunistic pathogen prophylaxis: *Cryptosporidium parvum* and *Pneumocystis carinii*. Laboratory Animal Science 49:331-334, 1999.

443. Ngo LY, Yogev R, Dankner WM, Hughes WT, Burchett S, Xu J, Sadler B, Unadkat JD, and ACTG 254 Team. Pharmacokinetics of azithromycin administered alone and with atovaquone in HIV-infected children. Antimicrob Agents Chemother 43:1516-1519, 1999.

444. Oz HS, Hughes WT, DNA amplification from nasopharyngeal aspirates in rats: A procedure to detect *Pneumocystis carinii*. Microbial Pathogenesis 27:119-121, 1999.

445. Vargas SL, Ponce C, Hughes WT, Wakefield A, Weitz JC, Donoso S, Ulloa AV, Madrid P, Gould S, Latorre JJ, Avila R, Benveniste S, Gallo M, Belletti J, Lopez R. Association of primary *Pneumocystis carinii* infection and sudden infant death syndrome. C.I.D. 29:1489-1493, 1999.

446. Hughes WT. Treatment and prevention of viral infections in patients with primary immunodeficiency diseases. In: Lederman H, ed. Clinical Updates in Primary Immunodeficiency Diseases. Englewood, CO: Postgraduate Institute of Meheim, Pub 1(3):1-6, 1999.

447. Abbasi S, Shenep JL, Hughes WT, Flynn PM. Aspergillosis in children with cancer: A 34-year experience. Clin Infect Dis 29:1210-1219, 1999.

448. Hughes WT. Pneumocystis. In: Strickland GT, ed. Hunter's Tropical Medicine and Emerging Infectious Diseases, 8th ed. WB Saunders, Philadelphia, Chapter 98, pp 701-705, 2000.

449. Hughes WT. *Pneumocystis carinii* pneumonitis. In: Behrman RE, Kleigman RM, Arvin AM. Nelson Textbook of Pediatrics, 16th ed. WB Saunders Co, Chapter 281, pp 1062-1064, 2000.

450. Hughes WT, Pizzo P. Infections in the compromised host. In: Behrman RE, Kleigman RM, Arvin AM. Nelson Textbook of Pediatrics, 16th ed. WB Saunders Co, Chapter 179, pp 780-788, 2000.

451. Hughes WT. Importance of clinical trials. In: Steen G, Mirro J, eds. St. Jude Children's Research Hospital Handbook of Childhood Cancer: A Handbook from St. Jude Children's Research Hospital. Perseus Press, pp 175-183, 2000.

452. Vargas SL, Ponce C, Gigliotti F, Ulloa AV, Prieto S, Munoz MP, Hughes WT. Transmission of *Pneumocystis carinii* DNA from a patient with *P. carinii* pneumonia to immunocompetent contact health care workers. J Clin Microbiol 38:1536-1538, 2000.

453. Hughes WT, Shenep JL, Rodman JH, Fridland A, Willoughby R, Blanchard S, Purdue L, Coakley DF, Cundy KC, Culnane M,

Zimmer B, Burchett S, Read JS, and the Pediatric AIDS Clinical Trials Group. Single dose pharmacokinetics and safety of the oral antiviral compound adefovir (bis-POM PMEA) in children with HIV-1 infection. Antimicrob Agents Chemother 44:1041-1046, 2000.

454. Hughes WT, Flynn B, Williams B. Nosocomial infections in patients with neoplastic diseases. In: Mayhall G, ed. Hospital Epidemiology and Infection Control, 2nd ed. Williams and Wilkins Co. , 1999.

455. Hughes WT. *Pneumocystis carinii*. In: Schlossberg D, ed. Current Therapy in Infectious Disease, 2nd ed. Philadelphia: Mosby Inc, Chapter 180, pp 684-685, 2001.

456. Hughes WT. *Pneumocystis carinii* pneumonia. In: Rudolph AM, Rudolph CD, Siegel NJ, Lister G, Hostetter MK. Rudolph's Pediatrics, 21st ed. McGraw Hill, New York, pp 1144-45, 2003..

457. Hughes WT. Pneumocystosis. In: Rondanelli EG, ed. Treatise on therapy and prophylaxis of infectious diseases. (in press).

458. Hughes WT. *Pneumocystis carinii* pneumonia. In: Stockman JA, Lohr JA, eds. Essence of Office Pediatrics. WB Saunders, Philadelphia, pp 318, 2001.

459. Oz HS, Hughes WT. Search for *Pneumocystis carinii* DNA in upper and lower respiratory tract secretions of humans. Diagnostic Microbiol Infect Dis 37:161-164, 2000.

460. Hughes WT. Mycobacterial infection in bone marrow transplant recipients (Editorial). Biol Blood Bone Marrow Transplant 6:359-360, 2000..

461. Oz HS, Hughes WT, Rehg JE, Thomas FK. Effect of CD40 ligand and other immunomodulators on *Pneumocystis carinii* infection in the rat model. Microbial Pathogenesis 29:187-190, 2000.

462. Hughes WT. <u>The Yellow Martyrs</u>. Writers Club Press (iuniverse. com), New York, pp 1-301, 2000.

463. Oz HS, Hughes WT, Varilek GW. A rat model for combined *Trypanosoma cruzi* and *Pneumocystis carinii* infection. Microb Pathogenesis 29:363-365, 2000.

464. Vargas SL, Hughes WT, Santolaya ME, Ulloa AV, Ponce CA, Cabrera CE, Cumsille F, Gigliotti F. Search for primary infection by *Pneumocystis carinii* in a cohort of normal, healthy infants. Clin Infect Dis 32:855-861, 2001.

465. Shenep JL, Flynn PM, Baker DK, Hetherington SV, Hudson MM, Hughes WT, Patrick CC, Roberson PK, Sandlund JT, Santana VM, Sixbey JW, Slobod KS. Oral cefixime is similar to intravenous antibiotics in the empirical treatment of febrile neutropenic children with cancer. Clin Infect Dis 32:36-43, 2001.

466. Hughes WT. *Pneumocystis carinii* pneumonitis. In: Burg FD, Gershon A, Ingelfinger JR, Polin RA, eds. Current Pediatric Therapy, 17th ed. Philadelphia: WB Saunders Co., pp183-185, 2002.

467. Hughes WT. Treatment of *Pneumocystis carinii* pneumonia. Advance for Managers of Respiratory Care. Marion Publication, Inc., King of Prussia, PA 10(1):51-52, January 2001.

468. van de Poll MEC, Relling MV, Schuetz EG, Harrison PL, Hughes WT, Flynn PM. The effect of atovaquone on etoposide pharmacokinetics in children with acute lymphoblastic leukemia. Cancer Chemother Pharmacol 47:467-472, 2001.

469. Hughes WT. Use of antimicrobial agents for treatment of infection in the neutropenic immunocompromised patient. In: Ricks RC, Berger ME, O'Hara FM, eds. The Medical Basis for Radiation Accident Preparedness. The Parthenon Pub. Bocca Raton, pp. 117-129, 2002.

470. Hughes WT. *Pneumocystis carinii*. Semin Pediatr Infect Dis 12: 309-314, 2001.

471. Ligon BL. Walter T. Hughes: Leader in the battle against *Pneumocystis carinii* pneumonia. (Biography) Semin Pediatr Infect Dis 12: 323-333, Oct., 2001.

472. Hughes WT, Armstrong D, Bodey GP, Bow EJ, Brown AE, Calandra T, Feld R, Pizzo P, Rolston KVI, Shenep JL, Young LS. 2002 Guidelines for the use of antimicrobial agents in neutropenic patients with cancer. Clin Infect Dis 34: 730-751, Mar 15, 2002.

473. Hughes WT, Armstrong D, Bodey GP, Bow EJ, Brown AE, Calandra T, Feld R, Pizzo P, Rolston KVI, Shenep JL, Young LS. Reply to "Lipid formulation of amphotericin B for empirical therapy of fever and neutropenia. (letter to editor) Clin Infect Dis 35:897-898, 2002.

474. Oz H, Hughes WT, Thomas EK, McClain CJ. Effects of immunomodulators on acute *Trypanosoma cruzi* infection in mice. Med Sci Monit 2002: 8(6): BR 208-211.

475. Hughes WT. *Pneumocystis carinii* vs *Pneumocystis jiroveci*: another misnomer. Emerg Infect Dis. Emerg Infect Dis 2003; 9: 276-277.

476. Oz HS, Hughes WT, Varilek GW. Provocative effects of immunosuppressants rapamycin, tacrolimus and dexamethasone

on *Pneumocystis carinii* pneumonitis in contrast to anti-PCP effects of mycophenolate mofetil. Transplantation 2001; 72: 9: 1464-1465.

477. Hughes WT. *The Last Leaf*, Writers' Club Press, New York, pp. 244, 2003.

478. Hughes WT, Flynn PM. Candidiasis. In: Feigan RD, Cherry JD, Demmler GJ, Kaplan S, eds. Textbook of Pediatric Infectious Diseases, 5th ed. Philadelphia: WB Saunders Co., pp. 2569-2579, 2004.

479. Hughes WT. Cryptococcosis. In: Feigan RD, Cherry JD, Demmler GJ, Kaplan S, eds. Textbook of Pediatric Infectious Diseases, 5th ed. Philadelphia: WB Saunders Co., 2602-2607, 2004.

480. Hughes WT. *Pneumocystis carinii* pneumonia. In: Feigan RD, Cherry JD, Demmler GJ, Kaplan S, eds. Textbook of Pediatric Infectious Diseases, 5th ed. Philadelphia: WB Saunders Co., pp. 2773-2782, 2004.

481. Hughes WT. *Pneumocystis carinii*. In Behrman RE, et al, eds. Nelson Textbook of Pediatrics, 17th ed. W.B. Saunders Co., Philadelphia, pp. 1154-1155, 2004.

482. Hughes WT. *Pneumocystis carinii* pneumonia. In: Gorbach SL, Blacklow NR, Bartlett JG, eds. Infectious Diseases, 3rd ed. Baltimore, MD: Lippincott, Williams & Wilkins , pp. 2339-2341, 2004..

483. Hughes WT. *Pneumocystis carinii* pneumonia. In: Gorbach SL, Blacklow NR, Bartlett JG, eds. Infectious Diseases, 3rd ed. Baltimore, MD: Lippincott, Williams & Wilkins , pp. 508-512, 2004..

484. Hughes WT. (Book Review). Dionisio, D et al. *Textbook-Atlas of Intestinal Infections in AIDS.* N Engl J Med 2004; 350: 1267-1268. , Mar. 18, 2004.

485. Hughes WT. *Pneumocystis carinii*: historical overview. In, Walzer PD, Cushion M, eds Pneumocystis Pneumonia. 3rd ed, Lung Biology in Health and Disease, vol. 194, Marcel Dekker, New York, pp 1-37, 2005

485. Hughes WT. Pneumocystis pneumonia in non-HIV infected patients: Update. In Walzer PD, Cushion, eds Pneumocystis Pneumonia. 3rd ed, Lung Biology in Health and Disease vol. 194, Marcel Dekker, New York , pp. 407-434, 2005.

487. Hughes WT, Dankner WM, Yogev R, Huang S, Paul ME, Flores MA, Kline MW, Wei L-J and PACTG Team. Comparison of atovaquone and azithromycin to trimethoprim-sulfamethoxazole in the prevention of serious bacterial infections in children with human immunodeficiency virus infection. Clin. Infect. Dis. 40: 136-145, 2005.

488. Hughes WT. The Pediatrician as Intravenous Expert. In, Baker JP, Pearson HA, eds. Dedicated to the Health of All Children. Amer. Acad. Pediatr. Evanston Ill., pp 156-157, 2005.

489. Nachman S, Gona P, Dankner W, Weinberg A, Yogev R, Gershon A, Rathore M, Reed JS, Huang S, Elgie C, Hudgens K, Hughes W. The rate of serious bacterial infections among HIV-infected children with immune reconstitution who have discontinued opportunistic infection prophylaxis. Pediatr 115:e488-494, 2005.

490. Hughes WT. The Seo article reviewed: Infectious complications of lung cancer. Oncology 19: 199-200, 2005.

491. Hughes WT. Bloodstream infections in cancer patients (Editorial) Eur. J. Cancer 41:1370-1371, 2005.

492. Weinberg A, Gona P, Nachman SA, Defechereux P, Yogev R, Hughes W, Wara D, Spector SA, Read J, Elgie C, Cooper M, Dankner W and PACTG Team. Antibody responses to hepatitis A virus vaccine among HIV-infected children with evidence of immunologic reconstitution on retroviral therapy. J. I. D. 193: 302-311, 2006.

493. Hughes WT. Should prophylactic antibiotics be used in afebrile neutropenic oncology patients? Nature Clin Pract Oncol 3: 130-131, 2006.

494. Hughes WT. Pneumocystis carinii versus Pneumocystis jirovecii (jiroveci) Frenkel. (Correspondence) C. I. D. 42: 1211-1212, 2006.

495. Hughes WT: **Ghosts of Misery Island**, Publish America LLD, Baltimore, 2006 (novel).

496. Hughes WT: Pneumocystis pneumonia. Chapter 178, In **Clinical Infectious Diseases**, Schlossberg, D ed., 3rd ed. Cambridge University Press, New York, pp. 1229-1232.

497. Hughes WT. Pneumocystis Pneumonia. In **Textbook of Pediatric Infectious Diseases**, 6th ed., Feigin RD, Cherry JD, Demmler G, Kaplan SL. eds., Saunders Elsevier Co., Philadelphia pp. 1271-1281, 2009..

498. Hughes WT. Aspergillosis. Chapter 210. In McMillan JA, DeAngelis CD, Feigin RD, Warshaw JB, eds. *Oski's Pediatrics: Principles and Practice,* 4th ed, Lippincott Williams and Wilkins, Philadelphia, pp.1301-3, 2006.

499. Hughes WT. Cryptosporidiosis. Chapter 218, In McMillan JA, DeAngelis CD, Feigin RD, Warshaw JB, eds. *Oski's Pediatrics: Principles and Practice*, 4th ed, Lippincott, Williams and Wilkins, Philadelphia, pp. 1327-9, 2006.

500. Hughes WT. Candidiasis. Chapter 208, In McMillan JA, DeAngelis CD, Feigin RD, Warshaw JB, eds. *Osk's Pediatrics: Principles and Practice,* 4th ed, Lippincott, Williams and Wilkins, Philadelphia, pp. 1294-7, 2006.

501. Madden RM, Pui CH, Hughes WT, Flynn PM, Leung W. Prophylaxis of Pneumocystis carinii pneumonia with ato-vaquone in children with leukemia. Cancer. 2007, 109: 1654-1658.

503. Hughes WT. Transmission of Pneumocystis sp. Among renal transplant recipients (editorial) Clin Infect Dis . 2007; 44: 1150-1.

504. Hughes WT. ***Suffer the Little Children.*** (Novel) Publish America LLD, Baltimore, MD, 2011, 297 p.

505. McCullers JA, Williams BF, Wu S, Smeltzer M, Williams BG, Hayden RT, Howard SC, Pui CH, Hughes WT. Health care-associated infections at a children's cancer hospital, 1983-2008. J. Pediatr Infect Dis Soc, vol 1:26-34, 2012.

Abstracts

1. Hughes WT, Falkner F. Measurement of mycotic colony growth by planimetry. (Proceedings SSPR). South Med J 58:1585, 1965.

2. Hughes WT. Chromoblastomycosis: Successful treatment with topical amphotericin B. (Proceedings SSPR). South Med J 59:1369, 1966.

3. Hughes WT, Kim MY. In vitro survival of Candida albicans in urine. (Proceedings SSPR). South Med J 59:1369, 1966.

4. Hughes WT, Kim MY, Rathauser V. A histoplasmin tine test: Evaluation in 1070 infants and children. (Proceedings SSPR). South Med J 60:1365, 1967.

5. Franco S, Hughes WT. Systemic blastomycosis of childhood: A clinical and epidemiological study. (Proceedings SSPR). South Med J 60:1365, 1967.

6. Hughes WT, Kim MY, Feldman S. A relationship between fungiuria and bacteriuria. (Proceedings SSPR). South Med J 60:1365, 1967.

7. Smith J, Hughes WT. Reconversion of the histoplasmin skin test: Reaction with live-attenuated viral vaccines. (Proceedings SSPR). South Med J 60:1351, 1967.

8. Hughes WT, Franco S, Kim MY, Feldman S. Mycoflora and the ecological relationship of bacteria indigenous to man. (Presented to SSPR). South Med J 61:1329, 1968.

9. Hughes WT. The role of infection in leukemia deaths. (Presented to SSPR, Nov 1971). South Med J 63:1494-1495, 1960.

10. Hughes WT, Kim HK. Mycoflora in cystic fibrosis: Ecologic aspects of Pseudomonas aeruginosa and Candida albicans. (Proceedings SSPR and presented at V Congress of International Society for Human and Animal Mycology, University of Paris Faculty of Medicine, Paris, July 9, 1971). South Med J 63:1495-1496, 1970.

11. Hughes W. Disseminated mycoses in childhood leukemia. (Presented at XIII International Congress of Pediatrics, Vienna, Austria, 1971).

12. Hughes W. Effects of pentamidine isethionate in *Pneumocystis carinii* pneumonitis. (Presented at Interscience Conference on Antibiotics and Chemotherapy, Oct 1971).

13. Smith JW, Hughes WT, Kim HK. Characterization of *Pneumocystis carinii* by biophysical and enzymatic methods. (Presented at American Society for Microbiology, Minneapolis, Minnesota, 1971).

14. Kim HK, Hughes W, Feldman S. Studies of *Pneumocystis carinii* with fluorescein labeled antibody. (Presented at SSPR). Clin Res 10:103, 1972.

15. Hughes WT, Kim HK, Feldman S, Price R, Coburn T. *Pneumocystis carinii* pneumonitis. Society for Pediatric Research, Washington, DC, 1972.

16. Feldman S, Hughes WT, Darlington JW, Gravell M, Kim HK. Efficacy of Poly I: Poly C in the treatment of herpes zoster infections. Interscience Conference on Antimicrobial Agents and Chemotherapy. Atlantic City, 1972.

17. Hughes W. Infection problems in childhood cancer. Seventh International Cancer Conference, Los Angeles, 1972.

18. Hughes W. Infections during remission of acute lymphocytic leukemia. Late effects of Cancer Workshop, Boston, 1972.

19. Hughes W, Price RA, Kafatos AG, Sisko F, Havron S, Schonland M, Smythe PM. Protein-calorie malnutrition: A host determinant for P carinii pneumonitis. Soc Ped Res, San Francisco, 1973.

20. Cox F, Hughes W. Isolation of cytomegalovirus from feces and tears. Soc Ped Res, San Francisco, 1973.

21. Hughes W. Signs, symptoms and pathophysiology of *Pneumocystis carinii* pneumonia. Symposium on *P carinii* infection. National Inst of Health, Bethesda, MD, 1973.

22. Price RA, Hughes WT, Kim HK. *Pneumocystis carinii* pneumonitis: Pathogenic and host susceptibility. Pan American Meeting of Pediatric Pathology, Mexico City, 1973.

23. Hughes WT, McNabb PC, Makres TD, Feldman S. Prevention and treatment of *Pneumocystis carinii* pneumonitis. Soc Ped Res, 1974.

24. Price RA, Hughes WT, Sanyal SK. Histogenesis and residual pulmonary changes in *Pneumocystis carinii* pneumonitis. Soc Ped Res, 1974.

25. Sanyal SK, Hughes WT, Harris S. Acid-base profile and blood gas changes in *Pneumocystis carinii* pneumonitis. Soc Ped Res, 1974.

26. Sanyal SK, Hughes WT, Harris S. Continuous negative chest-wall pressure in the management of hypoxia in older children. Am Acad Pediatr, San Francisco, 1974.

27. Hughes WT, Feldman S, Sanyal SK. Trimethoprim-sulfamethoxazole in the treatment of *Pneumocystis carinii* pneumonitis. Soc Ped Res, New Orleans, 1975.

28. Hughes WT. Treatment of *Pneumocystis carinii* pneumonitis with trimethoprim-sulfamethoxazole. Wellcome Foundation Symposium on Combination Chemotherapy of Infectious Diseases. Toronto, 1975.

29. Pifer L, Hughes WT. Cultivation of *Pneumocystis carinii* in vitro. Soc Ped Res, Denver, 1975; Pediatr Res 9:344, 1975.

30. Sanyal SK, Hughes WT, Harris KS. Prognostic implications of sequential changes in acid-base and blood gas profile in children with *Pneumocystis carinii* pneumonitis. Soc Ped Res, Denver, 1975; Pediatr Res 9:400, 1975.

31. Sanyal SK, Hughes WT, Harris SK. A new approach to management of severe hypoxia in older children with diffuse pneumonitis. Soc Ped Res 9:400, 1975.

32. Feldman S, Hughes WT, Chaudhary S. Idoxuridine therapy in children with cancer and varicella-zoster virus infection. Presented at the Antiviral Symposium, Palo Alto, 1975.

33. Feldman S, Hughes WT, Darlington RW, Kim H. Therapeutic efficacy of topical Poly I:C in localized herpes zoster. American Society of Microbiology, New York City, April, 1975.

34. Weiner LS, Hughes WT, Box QT, Dupree E. Recurrent *Pneumocystis carinii* in Type I Dysgammaglobulinemia. South Soc Ped Res Clin Res 24:70A, January, 1976.

35. Hughes WT, Feldman S, Chaudhary S, Ossi MJ, Sanyal SK. Comparison of Trimethoprim-sulfamethoxazole and Pentamidine

in the treatment of *Pneumocystis carinii* pneumonitis. Soc Ped Res 10:399, April, 1976.

36.   Sanyal SK, Mariencheck WI, Hughes WT, Harris S. A prospective longitudinal study of pulmonary function status in children surviving Pneumocystis carinii pneumonitis. Soc for Ped Res Abstract in Pediatric Research 10:467, April, 1976.

37.   Gunasekaran M, Hughes WT. Cyclic AMP phosphodiesterase of Candida albicans. 27th Annual American Institute of Biological Sciences Meeting, New Orleans, LA, 1976.

38.   Feldman S, Hughes WT, Chaudhary S. Antiviral therapy for varicella-zoster infection in children with cancer: Evaluation of idoxuridine (IDUR) Interscience Conference on Antimicrobial Agents and Chemotherapy, Chicago, October, 1976.

39.   Hughes WT. Infectious Diseases in Cancer Patients. XVIII Reuniao Anual de Cancerlologia II Encontro Dos Ex-Residentes Do Instituto Central, Sao Paulo, Brazil, 22-27, November, 1976.

40.   Cox F, Hughes WT, Pearson TA, Laneer J, Hess D, Williams B, Moore E, Elliott S. An evaluation of the effectiveness of "Peninsula Rooms" and standard isolation rooms in the prevention of hospital acquired infections in children in a cancer hospital. Assoc Pract Infect Control, Miami, 1977.

41.   Gunasekaran M, Hughes WT. Differentiation of Candida species of gas liquid chromatography. Second International Mycological Congress, Tampa, August, 1977.

42.   Gunasekaran M, Hughes WT. A simple liquid medium for chlamydospore formation in Candida albicans. Second International Mycological Congress, Tampa, August, 1977.

43. Hughes WT. The antibiotic and chemotherapeutic approach to unusual infections: Roundtable Amer Acad Pediatr, New Orleans, April, 1977.

44. Hughes WT, Kuhn S, Chaudhary S, Feldman S, Verzosa M, Aur R, Pratt C. Successful chemoprophylaxis for Pneumocystis carinii pneumonitis. Soc Ped Res, San Francisco, April, 1977.

45. Hughes WT. Unusual infections. Roundtable on antimicrobial agents, American Academy of Pediatrics, New Orleans, April, 1977.

46. Hughes WT. Pneumocystosis and toxoplasmosis in the compromised host. 10th International Congress of Chemotherapy, Zurich, September, 1977.

47. Hughes WT, Kuhn S, Chaudhary S, Feldman S, Verzosa M, Aur R, Pratt C. Prevention of *Pneumocystis carinii* with trimethoprim-sulfamethoxazole prophylaxis. 10th International Congress of Chemotherapy, Zurich, September, 1977.

48. Pifer L, Hughes WT, Stagno S, Woods D. *Pneumocystis carinii* infection: Evidence for high prevalence in normal and immunosuppressed children. Amer Soc Microbiol, New York, October, 1977.

49. Chaudhary S, Feldman S, Ossi MJ, Webster RG, Hughes WT. Serologic responses and adverse reactions to bivalent split influenza virus vaccine in children with cancer. Amer Soc Microbiol, New York, October, 1977.

50. Chaudhary S, Hughes WT, Feldman S, Sanyal SK, Coburn T, Ossi M, Cox F. Percutaneous transthoracic needle aspiration of the lung for the diagnosis of *Pneumocystic carinii* pneumonitis. XV International Congress of Pediatrics, New Delhi, October, 1977.

51. Hughes WT. Antibiotic therapy in infancy and childhood - An update. National Medical Association, Washington, DC, July, 1978.

52. Hughes WT. Childhood Pneumonia; New Infections; and Immunizations. Great Smoky Mountain Pediatric Seminar, Gatlinburg, TN, June, 1978.

53. Hughes WT. New Infections; Anti-Viral Therapy; and Immunizations. American Academy of Pediatrics, CME, No 7, San Juan, Puerto Rico, March, 1978.

54. Hughes WT. Trimethoprim-sulfamethoxazole. American Academy of Pediatrics, Chicago, October, 1978.

55. Hughes WT. Advances in supportive care: Infection. American Cancer Society National Conference on the Care of the Child with Cancer, Boston, September, 1978.

56. Hughes WT. Use of trimethoprim-sulfamethoxazole in the management of cancer patients. XII International Cancer Conference, Buenos Aires, October, 1978.

57. Feldman S, Wilber RB, Hughes WT. Impact of unstructured delivery of chemoprophylaxis for *P carinii* pneumonitis. American Society Microbiology, October, 1978.

58. Cox F, Coburn T, Hughes WT. 67 Gallium scanning for infections in children. South Soc Ped Res (New Orleans) 1978.

59. Yolken RH, Stopa PJ, Hughes WT. Rapid diagnosis of bacterial infections by the direct measurement of $_h$-lactamase in clinical specimens. Amer Soc Microbiol, Miami Beach, May, 1980.

60. Hughes WT. Statical effect of trimethoprim-sulfamethoxazole on *Pneumocystis carinii*. Soc Ped Res, Atlanta, May, 1979.

61. Hughes WT. *Pneumocystis carinii* infection in the compromised host. Amer Lung Assoc, Las Vegas, May, 1979.

62. Hughes WT. Current use of trimethoprim-sulfamethoxazole. Clinical Pharmacology Section. American Academy of Pediatrics, San Francisco, October, 1979.

63. Hughes WT. Acute lower respiratory tract infection; urinary tract infection; chronic lower respiratory tract infection; acute upper respiratory infection. American Academy of Pediatrics, CME No 7. Buena Vista, FL, December, 1979.

64. Stagno S, Pifer LL, Hughes WT, Brasfield DM, Tiller RE. *Pneumocystis carinii*, a cause of pneumonitis in young immunocompetent infants. 19th Interscience Conference on Anitmicrobial Agents and Chemotherapy, Session 99, Boston, October, 1979.

65. Hughes WT. Lung Infections in Patients with Cystic Fibrosis. Cystic Fibrosis Foundation Annual Meeting. San Antonio, April, 1980.

66. Hughes WT. "Management of the Febrile Neutropenic Patient" and "Pneumocystis carinii pneumonia". 17th Annual Infectious Diseases Symposium, Wilmington, May, 1980.

67. Hughes WT. Acute urinary tract infection, acute upper respiratory tract infection, chronic lower respiratory infection and acute lower respiratory tract infection. American Academy of Pediatrics, CME No 17, St. Louis, MO, 1978.

68. Hughes WT, Townsend TR. Nosocomial infection in the immunosuppressed child. 2nd Interstitial Conference on Nosocomial Infection. (Center for Disease Control). Atlanta, August, 1980.

69. Hughes WT. Pneumonitis in the immunosuppressed child. Amer Acad Pediatr Section on Chest, Detroit, October, 1980.

70. Hughes WT. Treatment and Prevention of Pneumocystis carinii pneumonia in children. Symposium on Trimethoprim-sulfamethoxazole. Cambridge, MA, November, 1980.

71. Stokes DC, Hughes WT, Alderson PO, King RE, Garfunkel D. Rat model of *Pneumocystis carinii* pneumonitis: Chest radiography and gallium-67 scintigraphy. American Thoracic Soc, Am Rev Respir Dis 123:162, 1981.

72. Stokes DC, Hughes WT, King RE. Rat model for *Pneumocystis carinii* pneumonia: change in lung compliance. Am Rev Respir Dis 123:163, 1981.

73. Hughes WT. Cytomegalovirus, herpes simplex and zoster in the oncology patient. Assoc Pract Infect Control, Baltimore, March 25, 1982.

74. Hughes WT. Semi-synthetic penicillin. Tennessee Medical Association, Memphis, April 15, 1982.

75. Hughes WT. Mode of acquisition for de novo *Pneumocystis carinii* infection. American Pediatric Society/Society for Pediatric Research, Washington, DC, May 13, 1982.

76. Hughes WT. Provocation of *Pneumocystis carinii* pneumonia with a T-lymphocyte inhibitor (cyclosporin A). American

Pediatric Soc/Soc for Pediatric Research, Washington, May 1982.

77. Hughes WT. Systemic candidiasis. International Soc for Clin Lab Techol and Amer Med Technol, Joint Convention Seminar. Nashville, August 14-21, 1982.

78. Hughes WT. Anti-infective therapy in the immunosuppressed patient. International Symposium in Development Pharmacology. Toronto, October 6, 1982.

79. Hughes WT. Prophylaxis and treatment of *Pneumocystis carinii*. 13th International Cancer Congress, Seattle, September 15, 1982.

80. Hughes WT. Tuberculosis today. Third National Pediatric Infectious Diseases Seminar, Las Vegas, February, 1983.

81. Hughes WT. Fungi: Friends and foes. Third National Pediatric Infectious Diseases Seminar, Las Vegas, February, 1983.

82. Hughes WT. Fever and Neutropenia. Third National Pediatric Infectious Diseases Seminar, Las Vegas, February, 1983.

83. Hughes WT. Ketoconazole and candidiasis. American Pediatric Society - Society for Pediatric Research. May 1983. Pediatr Res 17:272A, May, 1983.

84. Hughes WT. Histoplasmosis in the immunocompromised host. Amer College of Chest Physicians. 43rd Annual Meeting, Chicago, October, 1983.

85. Feldman S, Doolittle M, Hughes WT, Roberson P. Neutropenia in 60 children randomized to receive trimethoprim-sulfamethoxazole or amoxicillin for otitis media or urinary tract

infection. Interscience Conference on Antimicrobial Agents and Chemotherapy, Las Vegas, October, 1983.

86.   Hughes WT. Diagnosis and treatment of fungal and parasitic infections in children with malignancies. XVII International Congress of Pediatrics, Manilla, November 8, 1983.

87.   Hughes WT, Smith BL. Diaminodiphenylsulfone (dapsone): A new drug for *Pneumocystis carinii* pneumonitis. American Pediatric Society and Society for Pediatric Research, San Francisco, May 3, 1984. Pediatr Res (abstract 1090) 18:227A, April, 1984.

88.   Hughes WT. Special aspects of antifungal chemotherapy in children. Third International Symposium on Infections in the Immunosuppressed Host. Toronto, June 24-25, 1984.

89.   Hughes WT. *Pneumocystis carinii*: Biology and mode of trans-mission. 13th UCLA Symposium on molecular and cellular bi-ology on "Acquired Immune Deficiency Syndrome", Park City, UT, February 1984, Abstract. J Cell Biochem Suppl 8A, 1984.

90.   Sheehan RM, Stokes DC, Yeh Y-Y, Hughes WT. Alterations in lung lavage phospholipids in experimental *Pneumocystis cari-nii* pneumonia. Amer Thor Soc, 1984.

91.   Hughes WT. *Pneumocystis carinii* pneumonia: Chemotherapy and transmission. Amer Soc Trop Med Hyg, Baltimore, December 6, 1984.

92.   Hughes WT. Chemotherapy and trimethoprim-sulfamethoxa-zole vs. pentamidine. Symposium on clinical experiences with pentamidine, Chicago, March 28, 1985.

93. Hughes WT. Developmental therapeutics for *Pneumocystis carinii* pneumonia. International Conference on Acquired Immunodeficiency Syndrome. Atlanta, April 14-17, 1985.

94. Hughes WT. "Pulmonary infections in children" and "Childhood tuberculosis", Second Annual Pediatric Symposium, King Faisal Specialist Hospital and Research Centre, Riyadh, Saudi Arabia, April 24-26, 1985.

95. Gigliotti F, Hughes WT. Murine monoclonal antibodies to *Pneumocystis carinii*. 25th Interscience Conference on Antimicrobial Agents and Chemotherapy. Abstract 334, Minneapolis, October 1985.

96. Leoung GS, Mills J, Hughes W, Hopewell P, Wofsy C. Treatment of first episode *Pneumocystis carinii* pneumonia in AIDS patients with dapsone and trimethoprim. 25th Interscience Conference on Antimicrobial Agents and Chemotherapy. Abstract 830, Minneapolis, October 1985.

97. Hughes WT. Prophylaxis and therapy of pneumocytosis (non-AIDS). American Society for Microbiology (Seminar 213), Washington, DC, March 27, 1986.

98. Leoung G, Medina I, Hughes W, Hopewell P, Wofsy C. Dapsone is less effective than standard therapy for *Pneumocystis* pneumonia in AIDS patients. (abstract) Amer Thorac Society Meeting May 13, 1986, Kansas City, Am Rev Respir Dis 133:A184, April 1986.

99. Stokes DC, Gigliotti F, Snellgrove RL, Hughes WT. Experimental *Pneumocystis carinii* pneumonia in the ferrett. Amer Thorac Soc Meeting May 13, 1986, Kansas City, Am Rev Respir Dis 133:A184, April 1986.

100. Gigliotti F, Hughes WT, Davis D. Antigenic change on the surface of *P. carinii* induced by *in vivo* passive administration of specific monoclonal antibody. Soc Pediatric Research (abstract 910), Washington, DC, May 5-8, 1986. Pediatr Res 20:310A, April 1986.

101. Hughes WT, Smith-McCain BL. Effects of first generation oral hypoglycemic agents on *Pneumocystis carinii* pneumonitis. Amer Ped Soc/Soc Ped Research (abstract 921), Washington, DC, May 5, 1986, Pediatr Res 20:312A, April 1986.

102. Hughes WT. "Nosocomial infection in the immunocompromised host", Seminar on Nosocomial Infection in Pediatric Patients. Amer Soc Microbiology, Atlanta, March 5, 1987.

103. Hughes WT. "*Pneumocystis carinii* Pneumonitis" and "Antimicrobial prophylaxis in pediatric patients". Amer College of Osteopathic Pediatricians, Annual Meeting, Hilton Head, SC, April 23-27, 1987.

104. Hughes WT. "Pregnancy and active AIDS: the children" and "EBV infection in infants and children". First Annual Pediatric Symposium; Viral Diseases in Children. Humana Hospital-Audubon, Louisville, KY, May 8, 1987.

105. Hughes WT. "*Pneumocystis carinii* Pneumonia: an overview and update" and "Infection in the immunocompromised patient". Twelfth Annual Infectious Diseases Seminar, St. Paul Medical Center, Dallas, TX, May 20, 1987.

106. Hughes WT. "Pediatric medical education: An essential element in the children's hospital's commitment to excellence". National Association of Children's Hospitals and Related Institutions. Louisville, KY, October 1987.

107. Hughes WT. The immunocompromised pediatric patient. Seminar on "Aspects of epidemiolog in the pediatric patient". Research Medical Center and Ed Bixbey Institute, Kansas City, MO.

108. Hughes WT. New pediatric diseases. Seminar on "Aspects of epidemiolog in the pediatric patient". Research Medical Center and Ed Bixbey Institute, Kansas City, MO.

109. Hughes WT. Pediatric AIDS. "Review in Pediatric Infectious Diseases". (CME Seminar), Indiana University School of Medicine Indianapolis, October 28, 1987.

110. Hughes WT. Opportunistic infection in pediatric AIDS. National Institute of Child Health and Human Development. Workshop on Pediatric AIDS, NIH, March 30 - April 2, 1988.

111. Shenep JL, Hughes WT, Roberson PK, Blankenship K, Baker D, Meyer WH, Gigliotti F, Sixbey JW, Santana VM, Feldman S, Lott L. Double-blind trial comparing ticarcillin-clavulanate vs. vancomycin and ticarcillin in febrile neutropenic children. Amer Ped Soc/Soc Ped Res, Washington, May 1988, Abstract published Pediatr Res 23:382A, May 1988.

112. Gigliotti F, Ballow L, Hughes WT, Mosley B. Purification and initial characterization of a *P. carinii* surface antigen capable of inducing protective antibody. Pediatr Res 23:369A, May 1988.

113. Hughes WT. Chemoprophylaxis for *Pneumocystis carinii* pneumonitis with antifols. Seminar on "Infection in the immunocompromised host: Basic and clinical research issues". University of North Carolina and Burrough Wellcome Co, Research Triangle Park, NC, May 26-27, 1988.

114. Hughes WT. Animal models for *Pneumocystis carinii*. Society of Protozoologists. 41st Annual Meeting, Bristol, England, July 18-22, 1988.

115. Hughes WT. *Pneumocystis carinii* pneumonia: Experimental models. "Perspectives en infectiologie", Sociéte de Pathologie Infectieuse de Langue Francaise, Congrés de Faculté de Médecine, Lille, France, September 12-13, 1988.

116. Hughes WT. *Pneumocystis carinii*: advances in biology, pro-phylaxis and treatment. Seminar on Advances in Parasitology. Bracket Hall, London, April, 1989.

117. Hughes WT. Infection in neutropenia patients. International Congress on Strategies for Care in Oncology. Baltimore, MD, August 22-25, 1989.

118. Hughes WT. Prevention of *Pneumocystis* pneumonia (Recent Developments in *Pneumocystis carinii* infection). 29th Interscience Conference on Antimicrobial Agents and Chemotherapy, Houston, September 17-20, 1989.

119. Flynn PM, Marina N, Hughes WT. Disseminated *C tropicalis* in childhood leukemia: usefulness of computerized tomography. 29th Interscience Conference on Antimicrobial Agents and Chemotherapy, Houston, September 17-20, 1989.

120. Hughes WT. Progress in the management of febrile neutro-penic paediatric oncology patients. Symposium on Progress and Priorities in Childhood Cancer. Western Ontario London Regional Centre, The University of Western Ontario, London, September 28, 1989.

121. Hughes WT. Prevention of *Pneumocystis carinii* pneumonia. World Conference on Lung Health, Boston, MA, May 24, 1990.

122. Hughes, WT. Contemporary Issues in Infectious Diseases. Symposium on New Developments in the Management of Immunocompromised Patients. St. Johns Mercy Medical Center, St. Louis, MO.

123. Gutteridge WE, Pudney VS, Latter VS, Gray VL, Hughes WT. Efficacy of hydioxynaphthoquinones in experimental *Pneumocystis carinii* pneumonia. 7th International Conference on Parasitology, 1990.

124. Hughes WT, Kennedy W, Shenep J, Flynn P, Hetherington S, Fullen G, Lancaster D, Stein D, Palte S, Rosenbaum D, Liao S, Blum R, Rogers M. Safety and pharmacokinetics of 566C80, a hydroxynaphthoquinone with anti-*P. carinii* activity. 30th Interscience Conference on Antimicrobial Agents Chemotherapy, Atlanta, October 21-24, 1990, Abstract 861.

125. Hughes WT. Infectious Diseases and Oncology, National Conference on New Oncologic Agents. American Cancer Society, Dallas, TX, February 6-8, 1991.

126. Hughes WT. *P. carinii* prophylaxis. 6th International Conference on Pediatric AIDS, Washington, DC, February 10, 1991.

127. Hughes WT, Killman JT. Synergistic anti-*Pneumocystis carinii* effects of erythromycin and sulfisoxazole. American Pediatric Society/Society for Pediatric Research (Abstract 1030). Pediatr Res 29:174A, April 1991. (Presented in New Orleans).

128. Shenep JL, Adair JR, Roberson PK, Hughes WT, Flynn PM, Oakes L, Marina NM. Infrared, thermistor and glass-mercury thermometer body temperature measurement in children with cancer (Abstract 889). Pediatr Res 29:151A, April 1991.

129. Flynn PM, Hughes WT, Shenep JL, Crawford R. Disseminated fungal infection in children with cancer - a new look using computerized tomography (Abstract 823). Pediatr Res 29:140A, April 1991.

130. Hughes WT. Historical perspective of infection control practice. Assoc Pract Infect Control Annual Meeting, Nashville, May 5, 1991.

131. Falloon J, Hughes W, Land M, Lancaster D, O'Neill D, Dohn M, Greenberg S, Tuazon C, Rogers M, LaFon S, Labriole A, Lavelle J. 566C80 for the treatment of *Pneumocystis* pneumonia in AIDS. Am Fed Clin Res 1991.

132. Dohn MN, Frame PT, Baughman RP, Hughes WT, La Fon S, Smulian AG, Rogers MD, Brown N. Extended 566C80 therapy for *Pneumocystis carinii* pneumonia in AIDS patients. Internat Soc Protozol (Abstract no WS104), Bozeman, MT, 1991.

133. Hughes WT, Killman J. Macrolide-antifol synergism in anti-*Pneumocystis carinii* therapeutics. Internat Soc Protozol (Abstract no WS73), Bozeman, MT, 1991.

134. Hughes WT. *Pneumocystis carinii*: from Bristol to Bozeman. Internat Soc Protozol, June 1991.

135. Hughes WT. Interventional Antimicrobial Strategy: recommendation from the FDA. 17th International Congress of Chemotherapy, Berlin, June 1991.

136. Falloon J, Hughes W, Lancaster D, Land M, O'Neill D, Dohn M, Frame P, Greenberg S, Tuazon C, Rogers M, La Fon S, Labriola A, Lavalle J. 566C80 for the treatment of *Pneumocystis carinii* pneumonia in AIDS. VII International Conference on AIDS. Florence, Italy, June 16-21, 1991.

137. Hughes WT. Prevention of *Pneumocystis carinii* pneumonia. 2nd International AIDS Symposium, Morehouse School of Medicine, Atlanta, GA, September 5-7, 1991.

138. Hughes WR. *Pneumocystis carinii* pneumonia. Conference ofn AIDS-related apportunistic infection: developing effective therapies. Institute of Medicine, National Academy of Sciences, Washington, DC, April 9-10, 1991.

139. Vargas SL, Hughes WT. Substrate replacement limits *Candida albicans* gastrointestional overgrowth and subsequent invasions in neutropenic mice. XXXI Interscience Conference on Antimicrob Agents Chemotherapy. Chicago, 1991.

140. Hughes WT, Killmar JT. Synergistic anti-*Pneumocystis carinii* effects of clarithromycin and sulfamethoxazole. The First International Conference on the Macrolides, azalides and streptogramins. Santa Fe, NM, January 22-25, 1992.

141. Hughes WT. Prevention and treatment of infection; new drugs for the prevention and treatment of *Pneumocystis carinii* pneumonia. International Symposium Acute Leukemias. Münster, Germany, February 23-26, 1992 (Abstract). Ann Hematol (Suppl) 64:A119, 1992.

142. Hughes WT. New drugs for the treatment of *Pneumocystis carinii* pneumonitis. British Paediatric Immunology and Infectious Disease Group Annual Meeting, Coventry, England, 1992.

143. Hughes WT. Perspectives in infections of the immunocompromised host. (Guest lecture.) British Paediatric Association 64th Annual Meeting. University of Warwich, Coventry, England, 1992.

144. Hughes W, Leoung G, Kramer F, Bozzette S, Frame P, Clumeck N, Masur H, Lancaster D, Hyland R, Lavelle S, Safrin S, Sampson J, Weinberg W, Fallom J, Feinberg J, LaFon S, Rogers M, Sattler F, et al. Comparison of 566C80 and trimethoprim-sulfamethoxazole for the treatment of *P. carinii* pneumonitis. VIII International Conference on AIDS/III STD World Congress. Amsterdam, July 11, 1992.

145. Hughes WT. HIV treatment strategies for the 1990s (*Pneumocytis carinii*). Satellite Symposiums, VIII International Conference on AIDS. Amsterdam, July 19, 1992.

146. Hughes WT. *Pneumocystis carinii* pneumonia. Infections in immunocompromised host. Mississippi Infectious Disease Society. Natchez, MS, July 20, 1992.

147. Hughes WT, Vargas S. Air filtration prevents primary *Pneumocystis carinii* pneumonia in immunosuppressed rats. Interscience Conference on Antimicrobial Agents Chemotherapy. Anahiem, CA, October 12, 1992.

148. Hughes WT. Prevention of infections in patients with T-cell defects. Symposium on controversies in the management of infectious complication of neoplastic disease. Memorial Sloan-Kettering Cancer Center. November 18-20, 1992.

149. Hughes WT. Current therapeutic strategies in opportunistic infections of AIDS. American Chemical Society (205th National Meeting) April 1, 1993, Denver, CO, Abstract 162.

150. Hughes WT. Pneumonia in the immunosuppressed pediatric patient. Third Pediatric Infectious Diseases Seminar. Fitzsimmons Army Medical Center, Denver, CO, May 20, 1993.

151. Vargas SL, Shenep JL, Flynn PM, Pui C-H, Santana VM, Hughes WT. Azithromycin for the treatment of severe *Cryptosporidium*-associated diarrhea in two children with cancer. VI. Panamerican Congress of Infectious Diseases, Santiago, Chile, May 26-29, 1993.

152. Hughes WT. *Pneumocystis carinii* pneumonia. VI Panamerican Congress of Infectious Diseases, Santiago, Chile, May 26-29, 1993.

153. Hughes WT. Manejo de Infectiones del Niúo Neutrpénico. VI. Panamerican Congress of Infectious Diseases, Santiago, Chile, May 26-29, 1993.

154. Pagano G, Kennedy W, Weller S, McKinney R, Brown N, Hughes W. The safety and pharmacokinetics of atovaquone in immunocompromised children. IXth International Conference on AIDS, Berlin, Germany, June 6-11, 1993.

155. Hughes W, Jacobus D, Canfield C. Anti-*Pneumocystis carinii* activity of PS-15, a new biguanide folate antagonist. IXth International Congress on AIDS, Berlin, June 6-11, 1993.

156. LaFon S, Masur H, Sattler F, Frame P, Clumeck H, Hughes W, et al. The relationship of treatment-limiting adverse events to the time on therapy and plasma drug concentrations in a randomized trial of trimethoprim-sulfamethoxazole vs. atovaquone for the therapy of AIDS-related *Pneumocystis* pneumonia. IXth International Congress on AIDS, Berlin, Germany, June 6-11, 1993.

157. Hughes WT. Prevention of *Pneumocystis carinii* pneumonitis in infants and children with AIDS. CHI Conference on Prevention and treatment of Pediatric AIDS. Georgetown University Conference Center. Washington, DC, September 20-21, 1993.

158. Hughes WT. *Pneumocystis carinii* infections: current therapeutic and preventive measures. Annual Meeting American Academy of Pediatrics, Washington, DC, November 3, 1993.

159. Vargas SL, Hughes WT, Wakefield AE, Oz HS. Duration of *Pneumocystis carinii* persistance following *Pneumocystis carinii* pneumonitis. 47th Annual Meeting, Society of Protozoologists, Cleveland, OH, June 24-29, 1994 (Abstract p35).

160. Hughes WT. Update on the treatment of *Pneumocystis carinii* pneumonia. The New Jersey Infectious Diseases Society, 1994.

161. Hughes WT. Prevention of *Pneumocystis carinii* pneumonia. III. International Conference of Society for Hospital Infections. London, September 4-8, 1994.

162. Hughes WT. Comparison of atovaquone and trimethoprim-sulfamethoxazole in treatment of *Pneumocystis carinii* pneumonia. Symposium on Current Status of Mepron, at I.C.C.A.C. meeting. Orlando, FL, October 1994.

163. Hughes WT. Multiple opportunistic pathogen prophylaxis in children: atovaquone plus azithromycin compared with trimethoprim-sulfamethoxazole. Symposium on Current Status of Mepron, at I.C.C.A.C. meeting. Orlando, FL, October 1994.

164. Hughes WT, Killmer J, Oz H. Relative anti *Pneumocystis carinii* activities of ten drugs. Abstract (PB0621). Tenth International Conference on AIDS/International Conference on STD. Yokohama, Japan, August 1994.

165. Shenep JL, Flynn PM, Hetherington SV, Hughes WT, Patrick CC, Sixbey JW, Slobod KS, Roberson PK, Baker DK, Hudson MM,

Sandlund JT, Santana VM. Continued intravenous antibiotic therapy versus early switch to oral cefixime in neutropenic children with cancer and unexplained fever: A preliminary report. (Abstract). Infectious Disease Society America, Orlando, FL, 1994.

166. Hughes WT. Mother-to-infant transmission of HIV-1: new findings and therapeutic implications. VII Panamerican Congress on Infectious Diseases, Cartagena, Columbia, May 28-30, 1995.

167. Hughes WT. Controversies on antimicrobial prophylaxis in granulocytopenic hosts. VII Panamerican Congress on Infectious Diseases, Cartagena, Columbia, May 28-30, 1995.

168. Sillos EM, Hughes WT, LaFon S, Davis C, Woolley J, Studenberg S. Effects of disease and synthetic surfactant on absorption of aerosolized atovaquone in rats with *Pneumocystis carinii* pneumonia. American Thoracic Society, May, 1995.

169. Oz HS, Hughes WT. Acute fulminating babesiosis in hamsters with *Bahesia microti*: an experimental model. 70th meeting of the American Society of Parasitologists and 40th meeting of the American Association of Veterinary Parasitologists, Pittsburgh, July 6-10, 1995.

170. Oz HS, Hughes WT. Efficacy of atovaquone against *Babesia microti* infection in hamsters. 70th meeting of the American Society of Parasitologists and 40th meeting of the American Association of Veterinary Parasitologists, Pittsburgh, July 6-10, 1995.

171. Hughes WT. Atovaquone in the treatment of *Pneumocystis carinii* pneumonia. 3rd Congress of the National Association of Medical Parasitology, Brescia, Italy, 1995.

172. Hughes WT, Oz HS. Successful treatment of babesiosis with atovaquone. Thirty-fifth ICAAC, San Francisco, September, 1995 (#B52).

173. Patrick CC, Adair JR, Warner WC Jr, Church DA, Sanders RH, Krance R, Flynn PM, Hetherington SV, Hughes WT. Safety of ciprofloxacin as a prophylactic agent for prevention of bacterial infections in pediatric bone marrow transplant recipients. Thirty-fifth ICAAC, San Francisco, September, 1995 (#LM-17).

174. Vargas SL, Hughes WT, Silva AO, Bonoso G, Nachar R. Xylitol carbohydrate modulation of gastrointestinal flora. First International Pediatric Infectious Diseases Conference, Monterey, CA, September, 1995.

175. Vargas S, Hughes W, Wakefield A, Oz H. Eliminacion del *Pneumocystis carinii* del pulmon despues de una pneumonia por *P. carinii*. Accepted, XII Congreso Latinoamericano de Parasitologia, Santiago, Chile, October 21-27, 1995.

176. Hughes WT. *Pneumocystis carinii* pneumonia. 3rd Hong Kong International Cancer Congress, Hong Kong, November, 1995.

177. Hughes WT. Opportunistic infection in cancer patients. 3rd Hong Kong International Cancer Congress, Hong Kong, November, 1995.

178. Hughes WT. Opportunistic infection in cancer patients: An overview. Post-Congress Cancer Seminar, Beijing, China, November, 1995.

179. Hughes WT. *Pneumocystis carinii* pneumonia. XXVIII Meeting of Sociedal Chilena de Enfermedades Respiratorias, Valdivia, Chile, November 30, 1995.

180. Hughes WT. Pneumonia in the non AIDS immunocompromised host. XXVIII Meeting of Sociedal Chilena de Enfermedades Respiratorias, Valdivia, Chile, December 1, 1995.

181. Hughes WT. Advances in immunosuppressive treatment with impact on infections. XXVIII Meeting of Sociedal Chilena de Enfermedades Respiratorias, Valdivia, Chile, December 1, 1995.

182. Hughes WT, Kilmar J. Efficacy of sulfonamides alone in prophylaxis for *Pneumocystis carinii* pneumonia (abstract #572). 3rd Conference on Retroviruses and Opportunistic Infections, Washington, DC, January 28 - February 1, 1996.

183. Hughes W, McDowell J, Adams L, Flynn P, Hetherington S, Kline M, Shenep J, Yogev R, LaFon S. Evaluation of the novel nucleoside 1592U89 in a phase I safety and pharmacokinetics study in HIV-infected infants and children. 3rd Conference on Retrovirus and Opportunistic Infection (abstract #332), Washington, DC, January 28 - February 1, 1996.

184. Oz HS, Hughes WT. *Pneumocystis carinii* infection alters GTP-binding proteins in lungs (Abstract 761). Federation of American Societies for Experimental Biology, April 14-17, 1996.

185. Hughes WT. Nosocomial infections in bone marrow transplantation (Invited speaker). Society for Healthcare Epidemiology of America, Washington, DC, April 23, 1996.

186. Hughes WT. Pediatric AIDS. 8th Annual Pediatric Symposium, Saudi Pediatric Association, Riyadh, Saudi Arabia, May 1996.

187. Hughes WT. Opportunistic infections in the immunocompromised host other than AIDS. 8th Annual Pediatric Symposium, Saudi Pediatric Association, Riyadh, Saudi Arabia, May 1996.

188. Hughes WT, Killman J. Efficacy of intermittent doses of atova-quone and trimethoprim-sulfamethoxazole in the prevention of murine *Pneumocystis carinii* pneumonia. XI International Conference on AIDS, Vancouver, British Columbia, July 9, 1996.

189. Hughes WT. Therapeutic options for breakthrough PCP. (In Symposium on "Impact of Opportunistic Infections in HIV Disease.") XI International Conference on AIDS, Vancouver, British Columbia, July 1996.

190. Oz HS, Hughes WT. Effect of FK 506 in induction of *Pneumocystis carinii* pneumonitis in a virus-free rat mod-el (abstract 4). 41st Annual Meeting American Association Veterinary Parasitologists, Louisville, July 20-23, 1996.

191. Hughes WT, Armstrong D, Bodey G, Brown A, Edwards J, Feld R, Pizzo P, Rolston K, Shenep J, Young L. IDSA Practice guidelines: A progress report from the working committee on "Use of Antimicrobial Agents in Neutropenic Patients with Unexplained fever. 34th Annual Meeting of Infectious Diseases Society of America. Abstract I-51, New Orleans, Sept 18-20, 1996.

192. Oz HS, Hughes WT, Rehg JE. Efficacy of lasalocid against mu-rine *Pneumocystis carinii* pneumonitis. Abstract 286. 4th Conference on Retroviruses and Opportunistic Infections. Washington, DC, January 22-26, 1997.

193. Oz HS, Hughes WT, Rehg JE. A murine model for multiple oppor-tunistic pathogens: *Pneumocystis carinii* and *Cryptosporidium parvum*. Abstract 287. 4th Conference on Retroviruses and Opportunistic Infections. Washington, DC, January 22-26, 1997.

194. Dorenbaum A, Sadler B, Xu J, Van Dyke RB, Wei LJ, Moye J, McNamara J, Yogev R, Diaz C, Hughes WT. Phase I safety and pharmacokinetics study of micronized atovaquone in HIV-exposed or infected infants and children. Abstract 288. 4th Conference on Retroviruses and Opportunistic Infections. Washington, DC, January 22-26, 1997.

195. Hughes WT, Killmar J. Is trimethoprim of trimethoprim-sulfamethoxazole necessary for *Pneumocystis carinii* pneumonia prophylaxis? Abstract 289. 4th Conference on Retroviruses and Opportunistic Infections. Washington, DC, January 22-26, 1997.

196. Oz H, Hughes WT. Novel anti-*Pneumocystis carinii* effects of the immunosuppressant mycophenolate mofetil in contrast to provocative effects of sirolimus, tacrolimic and dexamethasone. Abstract 84. 72nd Annual Meeting of the American Society of parasitologists. Nashville, TN, January 24-28, 1997.

197. Shenep JL, Flynn PM, Hetherington SV, Hughes WT, Patrick CC, Sixbey JW, Slobod KS, Roberson PK, Baher DK, Hutson MM. Continuous IV antibiotics compared to oral cefixime in the empirical treatment of febrile neutropenic children with cancer. IDSA Satellite Symposium "Contemporary issues in infectious diseases." San Francisco, CA, September 15, 1997.

198. Ngoi LY, Yogev R, Daukner WM, Hughes WT, Xu J, Unadkat J. Pharmacokinetics of azithromycin when administered with atovaquone (abstract). Accepted, 5th Conference on Retroviruses and Opportunistic Infections. Chicago, IL, February 1998.

199. Oz H, Hughes WT, Rehg JE, Thomas EK. Efficacy of CD40 ligand and other modulators on *Pneumocystis carinii* infection

(abstract). 5th Conference on Retroviruses and Opportunistic Infections. Chicago, IL, February 1998.

200. Oz HS, Hughes WT. DNA amplification from nasopharyngeal aspirates in rats: A procedure to detect *Pneumocystis carinii* (abstract 10373). Experimental Biology meeting. San Francisco, CA, April 21, 1998.

201. Hughes WT. Clinical aspects of HIV infection. XVIII Congresso Panamericano de Pediatria, XI Congresso Latinamericano de Pediatria, XXXVIII Congreso Chileno de Pediatria. Santiago, Chile, April 27, 1998.

202. Vargas S, Latorre JJ, Ponce C, Weitz JC, Avila R, Lopez R, Beletti J, Gallo M, Madrid P, Hughes W. *Pneumocystis carinii* en pulmones de lactantes fallecidos en forma subita en sus casas versus lactantes fallecidos en el hospital. XVIII Congresso Panamericano de Pediatria, XI Congresso Latinamericano de Pediatria, XXXVIII Congreso Chileno de Pediatria. Santiago, Chile, April 28, 1998.

203. Vargas S, Prieto S, Muñoz MP, Ulloa AV, Ponce C, Hughes W. Portación asintomatica de *Pneumocystis carinii* en contactos immunocompetentes de un paciente on pneumonia por *P. carinii*. XVIII Congresso Panamericano de Pediatria, XI Congresso Latinamericano de Pediatria, XXXVIII Congreso Chileno de Pediatria. Santiago, Chile, April 28, 1998.

204. Flynn PM, Patrick CC, Baker D, Hetherington S, Hughes W, Santana V, Shenep J, Sixbey J, Brenner MK. Fluconazole prophylaxis in pediatric bone marrow transplant recipients: A randomized blinded trial. 9th International Symposium on Infections in the Immunocompromised Host. Assi, Italy, 1998.

205. Vargas S, Weitz J, Donoso S, Ponce C, Latorre J, Avila R, Benveniste S, Lopez R, Belletti J, Gallo M, Madrid P, Hughes W. An association of primary *Pneumocystis carinii* infection and sudden infant death syndrome (SIDS): A case control study. 36th Annual Meeting of Infectious Disease Society of America, abstract 747. Denver, November 1998.

206. Vargas SL, Prieto S, Muñoz MP, Ulloa AV, Ponce C, Hughes WT. *Pneumocystis carinii* person-to-person transmission from a patient with *P. carinii* pneumonia to immunocompetent contact healthcare workers. 36th Annual Meeting of Infectious Disease Society of America, abstract 85. Denver, November 1998.

207. Hughes WT. *Pneumocystis carinii* pneumonitis in patients without AIDS. American Thoracic Society and American Lung Association. Section on Clinical Controversies. Baltimore, October 18-19, 1998.

208. Hughes WT. *Pneumocystis carinii* pneumonitis. 2nd Michigan Pediatric Infectious Conference, Ann Arbor, MI, April 27, 1999.

209. Hughes WT. *Candida albicans*. Fourth Annual Infectious Disease Seminar. Driscoll Children's Hospital. Corpus Christi, TX, October 16, 1999.

210. Hughes WT. *Pneumocystis carinii* pneumonia. Second World Congress in Pediatric Infectious Disease. Manila, Philippines, November 2-6, 1999.

211. Vargas SL, Santolaya ME, Ponce CA, Ulloa AV, Cabrera CE, Gigliotti F, Hughes WT. Detection of *Pneumocystis carinii* DNA during mild respiratory infections in infants. 37th Meeting of Infectious Diseases Society of America (abstract 54), November 1999.

212. Hughes WT. *Pneumocystis carinii*: an emerging pathogen. VII Annual Meeting Sociedad Chilena de Parasitologia. Olmue, Chile, January 14, 2000.

213. Vargas SL, Santolaya M, Ponce C, Ulloa A, Cabrera C, Gigliotti F, Hughes WT. Infeccion por *Pneumocystis carinii* en una cohorte de lactantes normales. VII Meeting Sociedad de Parasitologia. Olmue, Chile, January 14, 2000.

214. Vargas SL, Ponce C, Hughes WT, Wakefield A, Waitz J, Donoso S, Ulloa A, Madrid P, Gould S, Latorre J, Avila R, Benveniste S, Gallo M, Belletti J, Lopez R. Asociacion entre primo-infeccion asintomatica por *Pneumocystis carinii* y sindrome de muerte sribita (SMS). Sociedad Argentina de Pediatria. October 21-23, 1999.

215. Dankner W, Yogev R, Hughes W, Xu J, The Pediatric ACTG 254 Team. Phase II/III, Randomized, double-blind trial to compare atovaquone plus azithromycin to trimethoprim-sulfamethox-azole in the prevention of multiple opportunistic pathogen infections (MOPPS) in HIV-infected children. Soc Pediatr Res – Amer Ped Soc (abstract 1531), Boston, May 13, 2000. Pediatr Res (Supplement) 47:260A, 2000.

216. Vargas SL, Ponce CA, Ambrose HE, Avendano LF, Contreras L, Gallo M, Belleti J, Lachsinger V, Benveniste S, Veloso L, Hughes WT. Association of *Pneumocystis carinii* and sudden infant death further documented by DNA amplification. (Abstract 479) 38th Meeting of IDSA, New Orleans, September 7-10, 2000.

217. Hughes WT. Nosocomial infections in the immunocom-promised host. XX Jornadas Pediatricias Conmemorativas, Nuevos Retos en Pediatria, and XIV Jornadas de enfermeria Pediatricia, Culiacan, Mexico, September 21-23, 2000.

218. Hughes WT. Immunization in the immunocompromised host. XX Jornadas Pediatricias Conmemorativas, Nuevos Retos en Pediatria, and XIV Jornadas de enfermeria Pediatricia, Culiacan, Mexico, September 21-23, 2000.

219. Hughes WT. Selected pharmacological aspects of anti-toxoplasma drugs in the brain. Symposium on Toxoplasmosis and Schizophrenia. The Stanley Foundation and the Johns Hopkins University School of Medicine, Annapolis, Maryland, November 15-17, 2000.

220. Hughes WT. Use of antimicrobial agents for treatment of infection in the neutropenic immunocompromised patient. 4th International Conference REAC/TS on "The Medical Basis for Radiation Accident Preparedness: Focus on Clinical Care." Orlando, Florida, March 6-9, 2001.

221. Hughes WT. Biological terrorism and the pediatrician. MS Chapter, American Academy of Pediatrics, Jackson, Mississippi, May 16-18, 2001.

222. Hughes WT. Histoplasmosis: An update. MS Chapter, American Academy of Pediatrics, Jackson, Mississippi, May 16-18, 2001.

223. \\\Weinberg A, Nachman SA, Huang S, White C, Yogev R, Hughes W, Wara D, Elgie C, Dankner W and PACTG 1008 Team. Antibody response to hepatitis A virus vaccine (HAVV) in immune recovered HIV-infected children on HAART. 41st International Conference on Antimicrobial Agents of Chemotherapy (ICAAC), Chicago, Illinois, September 22, 2001.

224. Oz HS, Hughes WT, Thomas EK, McClain CJ. Effects of immunomodulators on acute *Trypanosoma crui* in mice. The FASEB Journal. 2002: 16 (a600) 459.13.

225. Oz HS, Hughes WT, Kinde H. Successful cultivation of *Halicephalobus deletrix* from a horse kidney and in vitro drug discovery. FASEB J (Experimental Biology) 2003; 17(4): A688, abstract 408.2, Apr. 11-15, 2003.

226. Best VM, Capparelli EV, Elgie C, Yogev R, Hughes W, Dankner W and PACTG 254 Protocol Team. Population pharmacokinetics of atovaquone in pediatric HIV patients, Abstract 073; Amer. College of Clinical Pharmacol. Palm Harbor, FL, Sept. 19, 2003.

227. Dankner W, Nachman SA, Hughes WT, Gona P, Huang S, Elgie C, Yogev R and the PACTG 1008 Team. An observational study of the rate of opportunistic infection events in HIV-infected children who have demonstrated imunological reconstitution and who have discontinued OI prophylaxis. 11th Conference on Retroviruses and Opportunistic Infections. Abstract S-6, Feb 8-11, 2004, San Francisco.

228. Weinberg A, Nachman SA, Gona P, Defechereux P, Yogev R, Hughes W, Wara D, Elgie C, Cooper M, Dankner W and the PACTG 1008 Team. Antibody responses to hepatitis A viruse vaccine among HIV-infected children with evidence of immunologic reconstitution. 11th Conference on Retroviruses and Opportunistic Infections. Abstract S-29, Feb. 8-11, 2004, San Francisco.

INVITED LECTURESHIPS (Since 1981):

1981   National Institutes of Health, National Cancer Institute, Pediatric Oncology Branch, Bethesda, Maryland

1981   The Medical College of Wisconsin, Department of Pediatrics, Milwaukee, Wisconsin

1981   Tufts University, New England Medical Center Hospital, Department of Pediatrics

1981   University of Alabama Medical Center, Department of Pediatrics, Birmingham, Alabama

1981   University of Texas System Cancer Center, M.D. Anderson Hospital and Tumor Institute, Houston, Texas

1981   Wright State University School of Medicine, Dayton, Ohio

1981   College of Medicine and Dentistry of New Jersey, Department of Pediatrics, Newark, New Jersey

1981   The Johns Hopkins University School of Medicine, Department of Pediatrics, Baltimore, Maryland

1981   University of Pittsburgh School of Medicine, Department of Pediatrics, Pittsburgh, Pennsylvania

1981   Beth Israel Medical Center, Department of Medicine, New York, New York

1982   St. Christopher's Hospital for Children, Temple University School of Medicine, Philadelphia, Pennsylvania

1982   University of Texas Health Sciences Center at San Antonio, Department of Pediatrics, San Antonio, Texas

1982   University of Minnesota Medical School, Department of Medicine, Minneapolis, Minnesota

1982   St. Elizabeth Hospital Medical Center, Youngstown, Ohio

1982   Children's Hospital Medical Center, Akron, Ohio

1982   University of California, San Francisco, Department of Medicine, San Francisco, California

1982   Nassau County Medical Center, Department of Pediatrics, East Meadow, New York

1983   Baylor University College of Medicine, Department of Pediatrics, Houston, Texas

1983   Lovelace Medical Center, Albuquerque, New Mexico

1983   University of Michigan, Department of Pediatrics, Ann Arbor Michigan

1983   University of Arkansas for Medical Sciences, Arkansas Children's Hospital, Little Rock, Arkansas

1983   Montefiore Medical Center, Albert Einstein College of Medicine, Department of Medicine, Bronx, New York

1983   Vanderbilt University School of Medicine, Department of Pediatrics, Nashville, Tennessee

1983   Rutgers Medical School, Department of Pediatrics, New Brunswick, New Jersey

1983   Nassau County Medical Center, Department of Pediatrics, East Meadow, New York

1984   University of Alabama Medical Center, Department of Medicine, Birmingham, Alabama

1984   Louisiana State University School of Medicine in Shreveport, Department of Pediatrics, Shreveport, Louisiana

1984   The Mayo Clinic, Department of Pediatrics, Rochester, Minnesota

1984   Children's Hospital, Ohio State University, Columbus, Ohio

1984   Harbor - UCLA Medical Center, University of California Los Angeles School of Medicine, Department of Pediatrics, Los Angeles, California

1984   Medical University of South Carolina, Department of Pediatrics, Charleston, South Carolina

1984   University of Colorado Health Sciences Center, Department of Medicine, Denver, Colorado

1984   Nassau County Medical Center, Department of Pediatrics, East Meadow, New York

1985   The University of Texas Health Science Center, Department of Infectious Diseases and Clinical Microbiology, Houston, Texas

1985   University of Mississippi, Department of Pharmacognosy, Oxford, Mississippi

1985   King Saab University, Department of Pediatrics, Riyadh, Saudi Arabia

1985   King Faisal Specialist Hospital and Research Centre, Department of Pediatrics, Riyadh, Saudi Arabia

1985   University of Oxford, Department of Paediatrics and Department of Medicine, Oxford, England

1986   Nassau Co. Medical Center, Dept. Pediatrics, East Meadow, New York

1986   University of South Florida, Department of Pediatrics, All Children's Hospital, St. Petersburg

1987   Austin Children's Cancer Center, Austin, Texas

1987   Medical College of Georgia, Department of Pediatrics, Augusta, Georgia

1987   State University of New York, Brooklyn, Department of Pediatrics and Department of Medicine, Brooklyn, New York

1987   University of California, Irvine, Department of Pediatrics, Orange, California

1987   University of Texas Health Sciences Center, San Antonio, Department of Pediatrics, San Antonio, Texas

1987   Brooke Army Medical Center, Department of Pediatrics, San Antonio, Texas

1987   Wilford Hall Hospital, Department of Pediatrics, San Antonio, Texas

1987   Memorial Sloan-Kettering Cancer Center, Department of Pediatrics, New York, New York

1987   Kentucky State Medical Society, Louisville, Kentucky

1987   The Johns Hopkins University, School of Medicine, Department of Pediatrics, Baltimore

1988   University of Mississippi, Department of Pediatrics, Jackson, Mississippi

1988   The Nassau Pediatric Society, Long Island, New York

1989   Wesley Medical Center, University of Kansas at Wichita, Kansas

1989   Columbia University College of Physicians and Surgeons, Department of Pediatrics, New York

1989   Yale University School of Medicine, Department of Pediatrics, New Haven, Connecticut

1989   Staten Island Hospital, Staten Island, New York

1990   University of Alabama, Birmingham, Department of Pediatrics, Birmingham, Alabama

1990   University of Indiana School of Medicine, Departments of Pathology and Pediatrics, Indianapolis, Indiana

1990   Memorial Sloan Kettering Cancer Hospital, Department of Medicine, New York

1990   St. Lukes-Roosevelt Hospital, Department of Medicine, New York

1990   San Francisco AIDS Foundation, San Francisco, California

1991   Harvard Medical School, Department of Medicine, Boston, Massachusetts

1991   North Shore Hospital, Cornell University Medical School, Department of Pediatrics, New York

1991   National Institutes of Health, N.C.I. and N.I.A.I.D., Grand Rounds, Bethesda, Maryland

1991   Robert Woods Johnson Medical School, Department of Pediatrics, New Brunswick, New Jersey

1993   University of Texas, Children's Hospital, Dallas, Texas

1993   University of New Mexico, Department of Medicine and Veterans Administration Hospital, Albuquerque, New Mexico

1993   University of Texas at Dallas, Department of Pediatrics, Children's Hospital, Dallas, Texas

1993   Presbyterian Hospital, Department of Medicine, Dallas, Texas

1993   St. Joseph's Hospital, Department of Medicine, Chicago, Illinois

1993   Northwestern University Medical Center, Department of Medicine, Chicago, Illinois

1993   Calvo McKenna Hospital, Department of Pediatrics, University of Chile, Santiago, Chile

1993   University of Rochester School of Medicine, Department of Pediatrics, Rochester, New York

1993   Harvard Medical School, Dept. Pediatrics, Children's Hospital, Boston.

1994   Medical College of Ohio, Toledo.

1995   University of Louisville School of Medicine, Louisville, Kentucky

1995   Driscoll Children's Hospital, Corpus Christi, Texas

1995   Department of Pediatrics, University of Chile, Santiago

1995   Department of Pediatrics, James Quillan Medical School, ETSU, Johnson City, Tennessee

1995   Department of Pediatrics, St. Vincent's Hospital, New York

1996   Department of Pediatrics, University of Indiana Medical School

1996   Department of Pediatrics, King Faisal Specialist Hospital, Riyadh, Saudi Arabia

1996   Department of Pediatrics, King Saud University, Saudi Arabia

1996   Medical and Surgical Staff, National Guard Hospital, Riyadh, Saudi Arabia

1997   Department of Medicine, Audie Murphy Veterans Administration Hospital, University of Texas, San Antonio

1998   Department of Pediatrics, University of Iowa, Iowa City

1999   Department of Pediatrics, Michigan State University, Kalamazoo, Michigan

2000   Faculty of Medicine, University of Chile, Santiago, Chile

2004   Hollings Cancer Center, Medical University of South Carolina, Charleston, SC

2004   Division of Infectious Diseases, M.D. Anderson Cancer Center, Houston, TX

NAMED LECTURESHIPS: (Since 1980)

1980   John I. Perlstein Memorial Lectureship, University of Louisville School of Medicine, Louisville, Kentucky

1981   William N. Creasy Visiting Professorship, University of North Carolina, Chapel Hill, North Carolina

1982   Sydney S. Moyer Memorial Lecture, St. Elizabeth's Medical Center, Youngstown, Ohio

1983   Allan Coopersmith Lectureship, 1983; The Johns Hopkins University School of Medicine, Baltimore, Maryland

1984   Frank Stevenson Visiting Professor of Pediatrics, University of Cincinnati School of Medicine, Department of Pediatrics, Cincinnati, Ohio

1986   Warren Wheeler Lecture, University of Kentucky Medical Center, Lexington, Kentucky

1986   Praxis Visiting Professor and Lectureship, St. Louis University Medical Center, St. Louis, Missouri

1989   Wellcome Visiting Professor, Robert Wood Johnson Medical School, UMDNJ, New Brunswick

1990   Ronnie Moss Lecture, Northwestern University, Department of Pediatrics, Children's Memorial Hospital, Chicago, Illinois

1991   5th Visiting Professor for the Annual Medical Board, North Shore Hospital, Cornell University Medical School, New York

1992   Lori Haker Lecture, Medical College of Wisconsin, Milwaukee

1993 Huésped Professor, University of Austral, Valdivia, Chile

1995 Wyeth Visiting Professorship, University of Hong Kong

1996 Pfizer Visiting Professorship, Vanderbilt University Medical Center, Nashville, Tennessee

1997 Russell Blattner Lecture, Baylor College of Medicine, Houston, Texas

1998 First Richard Bayley Lecture. St. Vincent's Medical Center, New York University, Staten Island, New York

2000 Penny Scurto Lecture, Louisiana State University School of Medicine, New Orleans

2004 Billy S. Guyton Lecture. University of Mississippi School of Medicine, Jackson, MS

2008 Gerald P. Bodey Lecture, M.D. Anderson Cancer Center, Houston, TX.

2112 Danny Thomas Lecture Series, St. Jude Children's Reserch Hospital Memphis, TN

INSTITUTIONAL COMMITTEES (in FILE)

EDITORIAL BOARDS: (Since 1981)

Pediatric Infectious Diseases, 1981-1991

Section Editor, Advances in Pediatric Infectious Diseases, Yearbook Pub., 1984 –1999.

<u>Journal of Acquired Immune Deficiency Syndromes</u>, 1988-2000

Editorial Consultant: <u>Report of the Committee on Infectious Diseases</u>, American Academy of Pediatrics ("Redbook"), 1991-1997

NATIONAL COMMITTEES: (Since 1981)

AIDS Research Advisory Committee, National Institute of Allergy and Infectious Diseases, NIH (1992-1995)

Committee on Infectious Diseases, American Academy of Pediatrics (1977-1983)

Advisory Committee on Anti-infective Drugs, Center for Drugs and Biologics, Food and Drug Administration (1985-1989), Chairman, 1989

Executive Committee Section on Infectious Diseases, American Academy of Pediatrics, 1990-1994

Pediatric Executive Committee, AIDS Clinical Trial Group, Division of AIDS, National Institutes of Health (1992-1998)

CONSULTANT:

BH PR/Vaccine Injury Compensation Program, Department of Health and Human Services (1989-1997)

Center for Drug Evaluation and Research, PHS, FDA (1989-1998)

Data Safety Management Board (DSMB), Division of AIDS, N. I. A. I. D., N. I. H., Bethesda, MD (2003-2007).

SOCIETY OFFICES:

President, Pediatric Infectious Diseases Society (1983-1985)

Executive Board, Pediatric Infectious Diseases Society (1980-1988)

Chairman, Committee on Infectious Diseases, Tennessee Academy of Pediatrics (1992-1997)

TEACHING: after 1981

1. Professor of Pediatrics, University of Tennessee Center for the Health Sciences, 1981-2004.

2. Lecturer in Pediatrics, The Johns Hopkins University School of Medicine, 1981-present.

3. Professor of Preventive Medicine, Division of Biostatistics and Epidemiology, University of Tennessee College of Medicine, Memphis, to 1991.

4 FEB 2015

St. Jude Infectious Diseases Faculty and Fellows: 1972-1998

FACULTY

Frederick Cox, M.D.
Sandor Feldman, M.D.
Patricia M. Flynn, M.D.
Arnold Fridland, PhD.
Francis Gigliotti, M.D.
Muthukumaran Gunasekaran, PhD.
Seth V. Hetherington, M.D.
Walter Hughes, M.D
Christian C. Patrick, M.D., PhD.
Linda Pifer, PhD.
Jerold E. Rehg, DVM.
Shyamal Sanyal, F.A.A.P., F.A.A.C.
Jerry L. Shenep, M.D
John W. Sixbey, M.D.
Karen Slobod, M.D.

R. V. Srinivas, PhD.
Shamala K. Srinivas, PhD.
Linda Toth, DVM, PhD.

FELLOWS WITH POSITIONS AFTER FELLOWSHIP

Sandor Feldman, MD	Billy Guyton Prof. of Pediatrics, Chief Div. Infect. Dis., U, Mississippi Medical Center; former Member St. Jude.
Frederick E. Cox, MD	Assoc. Prof. Pediatrics, Director Division Infectious Diseases, Med. College Georgia
Richard B. Wilber, MD	Executive Director, Clinical Research Coordinator, Brussels.
Subhash Chaudhary, MD	Assoc. Professor Pediatrics, Southern Illinois U, College of Medicine.
Sandra Elliott Johnson, MD	Private Practice, Louisville, KY
Douglas L. Bartley, MD	Chief, Pediatric Infectious Diseases, Maricopa Hospital, Phoenix, AZ.
Ho Kun Kim, MD	Private Practice, Tullahoma, TN
Haysam Tufenkeji, MD	Chair, Dept. Pediatrics, King Faisal Specialist Hospital & Research Center, Riyadh
William Malone, MD	Associate Professor Pediatrics, Geisinger Clinic, Danville, PA
Ellen Moore, MD	Assoc. Professor Pediatrics, Wayne State U. School of Medicine, Detroit.
Michael Ossi, MD	Director Clinical Research, Glaxo; Clin.Assoc. Professor Pediatrics, U. No. Carolina.
Michael Ryan, DO	Vice Chair Pediatrics, Geisinger Clinic, Danville, PA.; Clin. Assoc. Penn. U., Hershey.

Ricky Wilson, MD	Vice President, Syntax Labs., Inc., Palo Alto, CA (went to (CDC after St. Jude).
Patricia Flynn MD	Arthur Ashe Chair for Pediatric AIDS, Member, St. Jude; Prof. Pediatrics, U. Tenn.
Kelly Hendrickson, MD	Assist. Professor Pediatrics - Microbiology, Medical College Wisconsin, Milwaukee.
Kathleen Ryan-Poirier, MD	Assistant Professor Pediatrics, U. Florida, Gainesville.
Scott Henwick, MD	Assistant Professor Microbiology, U. Alberta, Edmonston.
James Lederer,	Asoc. Prof. Pediatrics and Medicine, U. Tennessee College of Medicine
David Issac, MD	Las Palmas Medical Center; Sierra Medical Center, El Paso, TX.
Jamie Fergie, MD	Director Infectious Diseases, Driscoll Children's Hospital, Corpus Christi.
Melisse Sloas, MD	Senior Clinical Investigator, Pediatric Branch Nat. Cancer Inst.; Assist. Prof. Pediatrics, Uniform Services University Health Services, Bethesda.
Sergio Vargas, MD, FIDSA	Professor Institute of Biomedical Sciences, Director Clinical Research and Pneumocystis Research Laboratory, U. of Chile School of Medicine, Santiago
Ross McCordic, MD	Deceased- during medical missionary service in central Africa.
Seema Abassi, MD	Private Practice, Memphis.
Ibrahim Al-Moshen, MD	Dept. Pediatrics, King Faisal University, Riyadh, SA.

Shari Orlicek, MD	Private practice, Amarillo, TX
Kathy Knapp, MD	Assist. Member, St. Jude Children's Research Hospital, Dept. Infect. Diseases
Karen Slobod, MD	Assoc. Member, St. Jude, Dept. Infectious Diseases
Johnathan McCullers, MD	Chairman & Prof., Dept. Pediatrics, U. Tennessee College of Medicine.
Steve Buckingham, MD	Assist. Prof. Dept. Pediatrics, Div. Infect. Dis., U. Tennessee College Med.
James Chodosh, MD	Dept. Ophthalmology, U. Oklahoma, Oklahoma City.
Brian Robbins, PhD	Dept. Infectious Diseases, St. Jude Children's Research Hospital.

CPSIA information can be obtained
at www.ICGtesting.com
Printed in the USA
BVHW091218130620
581303BV00001B/1

9 781478 753759